W9-BGM-805

Undertaking Sensitive Research in the Health and Social Sciences

Managing Boundaries, Emotions and Risks

FRESNO MEDICAL LIBRARY

Undertaking Sensitive Research in the Health and Social Sciences

Managing Boundaries, Emotions and Risks

Virginia Dickson-Swift

La Trobe University, Australia

Erica Lyn James

University of Newcastle, Australia

Pranee Liamputtong

La Trobe University, Australia

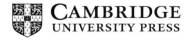
CAMBRIDGE
UNIVERSITY PRESS

CAMBRIDGE UNIVERSITY PRESS

Cambridge, New York, Melbourne, Madrid, Cape Town, Singapore, São Paulo, Delhi

Cambridge University Press
The Edinburgh Building, Cambridge CB2 8RU, UK

Published in the United States of America by Cambridge University Press, New York

www.cambridge.org
Information on this title: www.cambridge.org/9780521718233

© V. Dickson-Swift, E. James and P. Liamputtong 2008

This publication is in copyright. Subject to statutory exception
and to the provisions of relevant collective licensing agreements,
no reproduction of any part may take place without
the written permission of Cambridge University Press.

First published 2008

Printed in the United Kingdom at the University Press, Cambridge

A catalogue record for this publication is available from the British Library

Library of Congress Cataloging-in-Publication Data

Dickson-Swift, Virginia.
   Undertaking sensitive research in the health and social sciences : managing boundaries,
emotions and risks / Virginia Dickson-Swift, Erica James, Pranee Liamputtong.
      p.   cm.
   Includes bibliographical references and index.
   ISBN 978-0-521-71823-3
1. Social sciences–Research–Methodology. 2.   Medical sciences–Research–Methodology.
I. James, Erica. II. Liamputtong, Pranee, 1955– III. Title.

   H62.D4975   2008
   300.72–dc22

                                                                              2008014808

ISBN 978-0-521-71823-3 paperback

Cambridge University Press has no responsibility for the persistence or accuracy of URLs for
external or third-party Internet websites referred to in this publication, and does not guarantee
that any content on such websites is, or will remain, accurate or appropriate.

Every effort has been made in preparing this book to provide accurate and up-to-date
information which is in accord with accepted standards and practice at the time of publication.
Although case histories are drawn from actual cases, every effort has been made to disguise the
identities of the individuals involved. Nevertheless, the authors, editors and publishers can make
no warranties that the information contained herein is totally free from error, not least because
clinical standards are constantly changing through research and regulation. The authors, editors
and publishers therefore disclaim all liability for direct or consequential damages resulting from
the use of material contained in this book. Readers are strongly advised to pay careful attention to
information provided by the manufacturer of any drugs or equipment that they plan to use.

Virginia
For my mum who gave me an author's name in the hope that one day I would write a book

Erica
For all the people who have ever shared a personal story with a researcher

Pranee
To my two daughters, Zoe Sanipreeya Rice and Emma Inturatana Rice, who always put up with my writing

Contents

Preface

The impetus for this book came from the experiences Virginia had while undertaking a small qualitative project that investigated the impact of gambling on spouses and partners (Dickson-Swift, 2000). Gambling is a sensitive topic, and undertaking research on sensitive topics raises a number of particular methodological and ethical issues for both the participants and the researchers. When Virginia began interviewing the spouses and partners of gamblers it became clear that many of the participants who volunteered to be interviewed had not told their spouse or partner about their participation in the research study. For many of the participants, this interview was the first time that they had spoken to anyone at length about their partner's gambling and the effects that it was having on both them and their families. Many reported that participation in the research interview had forced them to think about the consequences of their partner's gambling.

Undertaking gambling research in a small town proved to be quite challenging. Virginia was not immune from the stigma that is often attached to those who have partners or family members who gamble. Many people wondered how Virginia came to be interested in gambling research that focused on the issues for spouses and partners. After the advertisements for potential participants were printed in the local paper, people began to speculate about her interest in such a topic. Some members of the local community concluded that her husband (quite a well known person within the community) must have had a gambling problem and that this was the reason behind Virginia's interest in this topic. Despite this not being the case, this illustrates one of the tensions that may be faced when researching on sensitive topics, particularly in small communities. When designing the research Virginia had not thought about the impact it might have on her or her family. Another unexpected dilemma was raised when Virginia encountered research participants in her day-to-day life, for example in the local supermarket. This raised the tension of balancing participant confidentiality while also behaving in a socially appropriate manner.

During the research interviews some of the participants became quite emotional as they retold their stories; others expressed fear, frustration, anger and sometimes resignation to the hopelessness of their situation. They often asked Virginia for advice about what they should do. Should they take a break from the relationship with the gambler? Should they take the children and get out of the relationship? Should they be seeking help? Should they stay and try to deal with it? While research was the main purpose of the interviews, Virginia found that many participants were expecting some advice. The project had been granted ethics approval from an institutional ethics committee, and throughout the approval process Virginia had considered that the participants might become distressed by taking part and may require counselling or support after participating. There were protocols in place for referring people to other agencies that could help them work through their problems; however, very few people were interested in those referrals. After the interviews were over many of the participants spoke of a sense of catharsis from the interview. They said it was nice to talk to someone and to 'get it off their chests'. This raised a dilemma for Virginia. Was this therapy? Were participants being given more than an opportunity to tell their story? In telling their stories, were they somehow changed by the process and, in listening to it, was the researcher also changed? Many questions about the nature of doing research on sensitive topics began to emerge.

Searching for the answers to those many questions proved to be difficult. After much reading of the literature it appeared that the 'story' of what doing research on a sensitive topic was actually like was missing from the published books and research reports. Many of the papers and books focused on the ethical issues of informed consent, gaining access and dealing with gatekeepers, but very few authors were telling the story of how doing research on a sensitive topic is not as straightforward as methods books may have you believe. Frustrated by the lack of researcher accounts of undertaking research, we embarked on a project to talk to researchers and record their experiences of undertaking research on sensitive topics.

In this book, we aim to tell the 'story' of undertaking research on sensitive topics from the perspective of those who actually do the research. The accounts of 30 researchers provided the basis for this book. The researchers we interviewed had a range of research experience, but all had been involved in research on sensitive topics. We chose the Monarch Butterfly for the cover of this book as these butterflies embark on incredible journeys across the world and are faced with many challenges along the way. For us the butterfly represents the challenges these researchers take and the journey across the world that their stories will take via this book.

In addition to the researchers' stories, we bring together a range of issues highlighted in the published literature to build a picture of what the experience of conducting qualitative research on a sensitive topic is like. Quotes from the actual researchers involved in the interviews are used extensively throughout the text (*in italics*) to illuminate the issues researchers face. We also outline some of the possible implications for researchers working in sensitive areas and recommend some changes to policy and research practice that will assist in the protection of researchers.

This book is written for researchers (both novice and experienced), transcribers, research funders, research supervisors, university risk managers and anyone interested in undertaking a research project on a sensitive topic. It aims to bridge the gap for researchers and to provide them with a resource that will assist them in their preparation for undertaking research on sensitive topics. It is also valuable for the training needs of postgraduate students who wish to undertake qualitative research on sensitive topics, as it provides essential reading regarding the risks and difficulties associated with this type of research. We hope that the content of this book challenges, guides and inspires you to undertake innovative qualitative research on sensitive topics.

Acknowledgements

Like any publication, this book would not have been possible without the assistance of many others. Firstly, we would like to express our gratitude to Nicholas Dunton, Senior Commissioning Editor of Cambridge University Press who has supported us throughout the development of the book. This book is based on empirical research that Virginia undertook as part of her doctoral project, which explored the experiences of researchers undertaking qualitative research on a sensitive topic. We are indebted to the 30 researchers who participated in the research interviews with Virginia. Their stories have allowed us an insight into the intricacies of doing research, which are often difficult to find, and we thank them for their contribution to this work.

We also thank our dear friend, colleague and mentor Sandra Kippen who has been an integral part of the team. Sandra was one of Virginia's honours and Ph.D. supervisors and as such over the years she has read many drafts of both her theses and this book, and has provided Virginia with ongoing support and supervision. Her wisdom and kindness are endless. We wish her well in her retirement.

We also thank our colleagues in the Department of Public Health at La Trobe University, Bendigo and Bundoora, who have supported us throughout the writing process. During the writing of this book Erica changed academic institutions. We thank Professor Afaf Girgis, and acknowledge the Cancer Council NSW for recognizing the relevance and importance of this topic and for allowing Erica to continue working on this book in her new role.

We wish also to acknowledge that earlier versions of the following chapters have been published elsewhere. Chapter 3 (Doing sensitive research: what challenges do qualitative researchers face? *Qualitative Research*, **3**(7), 327–353, Sage Publications), Chapter 4 (Blurring boundaries in qualitative health research on sensitive topics. *Qualitative Health Research*, **16**(6), 853–871, Sage Publications), Chapter 5 (Researching sensitive topics: qualitative research as emotion work. *Qualitative Research*, in press, Sage Publications) and Chapter 6 (Risk to researchers in qualitative research on sensitive topics: issues and strategies. *Qualitative Health Research*, **18**(1), 133–144, Sage Publications).

Finally, to our families and loved ones, we thank you for your encouragement and patience.

About the authors

Virginia Dickson-Swift has a PhD in public health and is a Lecturer in Public Health at the School of Public Health, La Trobe University, Bendigo, Australia. Virginia has taught across a range of units within both the undergraduate and postgraduate programmes. Virginia has particular interest in the role of emotion in qualitative research, and the use of qualitative methodologies in health research. She has published a range of papers based on this work internationally and presented her work at a range of conferences.

Erica James is a behavioural epidemiologist and a Senior Research Academic at the Centre for Health Research and Psycho-oncology (CHeRP), which is funded by The Cancer Council NSW and situated at the University of Newcastle, Australia. Erica's research programme emphasizes lifestyle behaviours and cancer control, including both qualitative and quantitative research with cancer survivors. She has published numerous papers and book chapters on various aspects of health promotion, methodological issues and teaching research methods.

Pranee Liamputtong is Personal Chair in Public Health at the School of Public Health, La Trobe University, Melbourne, Australia. Pranee has previously taught in the School of Sociology and Anthropology and worked as a Public Health Research Fellow at the Centre for the Study of Mothers' and Children's Health, La Trobe University. Pranee has particular interests in issues related to cultural and social influences on child-bearing, child rearing and women's reproductive and sexual health. She has published several books and a large number of papers in these areas.

Pranee has written and edited a number of research method books including *Qualitative Research Methods: A Health Focus* (with Douglas Ezzy, Oxford University Press, 1999, reprinted in 2000, 2001, 2002, 2003, 2004) the second edition of this book is titled *Qualitative Research Methods* (2005, reprinted in 2005, 2006 twice), and *Health Research in Cyberspace: Methodological, Practical and Personal Issues of Researching Online* (Nova Science Publishers, 2006). Her most recent method book is titled *Researching The Vulnerable: A Guide to Sensitive Research Methods* (Sage, 2007). She is now preparing three books: *Knowing Differently: Arts-Based and Collaborative Research Methods* (Nova Science Publishers), *Performing Qualitative Cross-Cultural Research* (Cambridge University Press) and *Doing Cross-Cultural Research: Methodological and Ethical Perspectives* (Springer).

What is sensitive research?

Efforts to address these issues would be enhanced by more published accounts of investigators' experiences in dealing with the effects on researchers of conducting studies on sensitive and emotionally laden topics: too little attention is given to documenting the process of carrying out research.

(Milling-Kinard, 1996:69)

In this introductory chapter we examine a range of different definitions of sensitive research. We discuss the historical developments of sensitive research and explore some of the sensitivities inherent in undertaking qualitative research on such topics. We outline the importance of researching sensitive topics and provide an overview of the remainder of the book.

Defining sensitive research

There are many definitions of sensitive research, ranging from those that refer to the topic of investigation to those that encompass the whole of the research activity, including its implications for practice and the wider research community. Joan Sieber and Liz Stanley (1988:49) define 'socially sensitive' research as, 'studies in which there are potential consequences or implications, either directly for the participants in the research or for the class of individuals represented by the research'. This definition of sensitive research is very general and by applying it, almost all social research could be defined as sensitive. All research has consequences of some kind. However, some consequences may be more directly harmful than others. Often discussions of what constitutes sensitive research focus too narrowly on only the ethical dimensions of sensitive research.

Raymond Lee (1993) argues that there are some advantages in defining sensitive research according to Sieber and Stanley's definition as it enables a broad definition of sensitive research to include some research areas that may not have been previously thought to be sensitive. However, he goes on to criticize the definition proposed by Sieber and Stanley, stating that it focuses on 'the consequences of the research rather than the specific technical and methodological issues that are inherent in sensitive research' (Lee, 1993:3). In order to develop a comprehensive understanding of the issues in sensitive research it is important to examine more than just the consequences of undertaking the research. Raymond Lee (1993) agrees that it is important to investigate the methodological issues as well, and to examine them from the perspective of both researchers and participants.

Previously, research on sensitive topics has been equated with research on those topics that are taboo (Faberow, 1963). Taboo topics are defined as those 'which are laden with emotion or which inspire feelings of awe or dread' (Lee, 1993:6). Claire Renzetti and Raymond Lee in their edited book *Research-ing Sensitive Topics* (1993:ix) define a 'sensitive' research topic as one that is 'intimate, discreditable or incriminating'. Health and social science researchers are involved in research being undertaken on a wide variety of topics that fit easily into either one of these definitions; for example, research exploring birth, death, cancer, grief, sexual abuse, violence, drug use or homelessness (Burr, 1995; Higgins, 1998; Kavanaugh & Ayres, 1998; Liamputtong Rice, 2000; Ridge, Hee & Aroni, 1999; Sque, 2000).

Lee (1993:4) puts forward another definition of sensitive research that encompasses the topic, the consequences, the situation and any number of other issues that may arise by saying that sensitive research is 'research which potentially poses a substantial threat to those who are or have been involved in it'. This definition is our preferred definition and the one that has been adopted for this book, as it suggests that sensitive research has the potential to impact on all of the people who are involved in it. This definition encourages us to examine the potential for harm to the researchers conducting the research as well as to the research participants taking part.

Lee (1993) proposes that sensitive research can be seen as threatening in three broad areas. The first of these areas is '*intrusive threat*', which deals with areas that are 'private, stressful or sacred' (Lee, 1993:4). Examples might include sexual or religious practices. The second type of threat is '*threat of sanction*', which relates to studies of deviance and involves the possibility that research may reveal information that is stigmatizing or incriminating in some way. An example of the threat of sanction might be conducting interviews with people with a drug addiction who may reveal illegal behaviours as part of the interview. The third type of threat that may be imposed by sensitive research is a '*political threat*'. This refers to the 'vested interests' of the powerful in society and in these situations researchers may trespass into areas that involve some sort of social conflict. An example of political threat can be seen in the work done by John Brewer investigating routine policing in Northern Ireland (Brewer, 1993). Raymond Lee and Claire Renzetti (1993:6) specify a number of areas in which some research is more likely to be threatening than others and these are summarized in Box 1.1.

Lee (1993:22) highlights that defining research that intrudes into the personal sphere as sensitive is not necessarily helpful because each person has a

Box 1.1 Areas in which research is likely to be threatening

(a) where research intrudes into the private sphere or delves into some deeply personal experience;
(b) where the study is concerned with deviance or social control;
(c) where the study impinges on the vested interests of powerful persons or the exercise of coercion or domination; or
(d) where the research deals with things that are sacred to those being studied that they do not wish profaned.

(Lee & Renzetti, 1993:6)

different 'private sphere'. This is well demonstrated in the published literature when we see that the topics and activities defined as sensitive vary widely across cultures and situations.

Some areas of personal life that researchers wish to investigate may not be so much private as emotional. For example, research regarding death and dying may not be private but may be emotionally taxing on those taking part in the research. Taking part in research of this nature may be a stressful experience for both the researcher and the researched and is therefore likely to be considered sensitive.

The threat of sanction can also be a problem for some participants in sensitive research as the participants may fear 'exploitation or derogation' by taking part in the study (Lee 1993:33). This is an important consideration for researchers studying sensitive topics who do not wish to exploit the community, for example, migrants, ethnic minority groups or low-income groups. Lee (1993:74) also states that 'research which might bring to light that which was formerly hidden' can be problematic for those taking part. The participants may face some sort of discrimination or stigma if a hidden part of their lives is revealed, for example problem gamblers or those with drug or alcohol addictions. When designing research on sensitive topics it is important to weigh the potential risks against the benefits by giving careful consideration to whether the research findings might further stigmatize or marginalize the population under study (Flaskerud & Winslow, 1998). There is a range of different methodological textbooks available to qualitative researchers undertaking research on sensitive topics and many of them document the issues faced by research participants (see for example Grbich, 1999; Liamputtong & Ezzy, 2005; Morse & Field, 1995). However, the issues faced by researchers have received little empirical attention.

Historical developments of sensitive research

The Chicagoans really were the first to carry out social research on sensitive topics and to give it some credibility. Many of the topics that were studied by the early Chicago sociologists would today be regarded as sensitive (Lee, 1993:11). Much of their research revolved around the family, friendships and communities and often involved gaining access to the private lives of the people taking part. Martin Bulmer (1984:90) points out, 'the Chicagoans were relatively unselfconscious about their methods, something which in part may have allowed them to sidestep the methodological and ethical issues raised by the study of sensitive topics'.

Social transformations of the 1960s and 1970s saw many changes taking place in social research across the world (Lee, 1993). Research programmes began to widen to include topics that had been previously paid little attention due to what has been termed 'perceived sensitivity' (Lee, 1993:13) for example, safe sex practices, domestic violence, alcoholism. There were other developments in social research, which included what has been described by Alvin Gouldner (1968, in Lee, 1993:14) as 'underdog sociology'. This type of research was associated with writers like Howard Becker (1963) who began to focus on researching the field of deviance.

Contemporary feminism has its roots in the political Women's Liberation Movement of the 1960s, which included campaigns against the objectification of women as sexual objects for male consumption and violence against women. Feminist research also emerged in the 1960s as a type of research, with arguments about whether or not there is a 'feminist methodology' (Stanley & Wise, 1993:176). Raymond Lee (1993) acknowledges that feminist researchers do tend to share a commitment to certain ways of researching women and their positions in society. There are some specific methodological traits of feminist research, which include the establishment of non-hierarchical relationships between the researcher and the researched (Finch, 1984; Oakley, 1981) and an acknowledgement of the subjective nature of research (Liamputtong & Ezzy, 2005; Stanley, 1990). Much feminist research seeks to understand the experiences of women in relation to such things as power, domination and disadvantage in gender relationships. In order to research and explain these types of issues much of the research focuses on the private experiences of the women. Some of the authors writing about sensitive research advocate for the adoption of some of the principles of feminist research to enhance research on sensitive topics (Campbell & Wasco, 2000; Jansen & Davis, 1998; Lee & Renzetti, 1993; Liamputtong, 2007; Renzetti & Lee, 1993; Ribbens & Edwards, 1998). An examination of qualitative research based on feminist principles uncovers a range of topics that are particularly sensitive, including rape (Bergen, 1993; Campbell, 2002), domestic violence (Ellsberg, Heise, Pena et al., 2001; Grossman & Kruger, 1999; O'Neill, 1996; Stanko, 1997; Taylor, Magnussen & Amundson, 2001), eating disorders (Kiesinger, 1998) and miscarriage (Swanson, 1999).

In order to undertake sensitive research it is often necessary to develop a relationship with those whom we are hoping to research. Sometimes this may involve the development of a personal relationship. This orientation of research is often emphasized by feminist researchers (Oakley, 1981; Stanley & Wise, 1991) who highlight the need to develop a special type of relationship with research participants in sensitive research. This type of particularly human relationship is a key element of researching sensitive topics and needs to be acknowledged. As Ann Oakley (1981:58) states, 'personal involvement is more than dangerous bias – it is the condition under which people come to know each other and to admit others into their lives'. This personal involvement is paramount in researching sensitive issues because of the often intimate nature of the research topics and the resulting subjectivity of the research process.

Sensitivities

As mentioned above, sensitive research encompasses research on a wide range of topics, undertaken in a range of different locations, using a variety of methods. There is no generic way to describe what sensitive research is. However, it can be characterized by examining some of the topics that may have been perceived as sensitive. Some examples of sensitive topics are sexual behaviours, deviance, drug abuse, death and other topics sometimes labelled as taboo subjects (Lee, 1993; Lee & Renzetti, 1993; Liamputtong, 2007). Many areas of research have the potential to be threatening to those taking part. Although there are some topics that are more obviously sensitive (such as those mentioned above), any topic could potentially be seen to be sensitive depending on the people being researched and their feelings about the topic. For example, the level of sensitivity of the topic may vary according to culture, age, gender or a number of other factors.

Topics that invade what has been termed the 'private sphere' (Lee 1993:5) are thought to be sensitive; however, there is a large variation in what people perceive to be private, and this varies across different ages, cultures and situations. The topic may also be sensitive because of the emotions evoked by participating. Joan Sieber (1993:18) refers to the 'perception of risk', highlighting that different groups of people will have different perceptions of risk. The gatekeepers, ethics committees, researchers and participants may all perceive the risk differently as this perception is highly subjective.

Other topics typically considered to be sensitive include those such as abuse, death and violence. It has been noted that there is the likelihood for research on these types of topics to evoke strong memories in the participants. Claire Draucker (1999) articulates her concerns when researching sexual violence. She argues, 'Of particular concern to violence researchers are the ethical implications of using procedures such as in-depth interviews and detailed questionnaires that may unleash painful emotions and memories in participants' (Draucker, 1999:162). The possibility that participating in research may 'unleash painful memories' has also been cited by Michelle Ramos (1989:59), who refers to this as the 'Pandora's box' phenomenon. It has been argued that often researchers do not adequately address the potential psychological harm that may result from research that evokes intense emotional reactions (Lee & Renzetti, 1993; Liamputtong, 2007; Ramos, 1989; Renzetti & Lee, 1993).

The importance of sensitive research

Whatever the definition, researchers need to undertake research on so-called sensitive topics to enhance the understanding of many of the issues that affect people in today's society. The decision to avoid research on sensitive topics could be seen by some researchers as evasion of responsibility. As Joan Sieber and Liz Stanley (1988:55) convincingly argue:

Sensitive research addresses some of society's most pressing social issues and policy questions. Although ignoring the ethical issues in sensitive research is not a responsible approach to science, shying away from controversial topics, simply because they are controversial, is also an avoidance of responsibility.

This point has also been made by Raymond Lee and Claire Renzetti (1993:10) who add that, in order to ensure that social scientists do not shy away from undertaking research on sensitive topics, they 'must confront seriously and thoroughly the problems and issues that these topics pose'. In order to confront the problems that research on sensitive topics may pose it is important to document the issues that this type of research can raise. While a small number of writers (Campbell, 2002; Johnson & Clarke, 2003; Lee, 1993; Lee & Renzetti, 1993) have attempted to document some of the challenges associated with this type of research, very few have focused directly on the issues that this type of research raises for the researchers. Much of the discussion in other researchers' accounts of sensitive research, focus mainly on ethical issues such as informed consent and the issue of harm. Kathleen Cowles (1988:163) highlights one of the dangers of focusing on ethics alone:

When the qualitative researcher delves into the private worlds and experiences of subjects, sometimes evoking strong emotional responses and sometimes pursuing thoughts that might otherwise never be revealed, consideration of the common ethical issues may not be enough.

There is a danger in focusing too narrowly on the ethical issues (although they are important). By narrowing the focus, the other issues inherent in sensitive research may not be given the consideration that they deserve.

Other researchers have illustrated that there are a number of specific theoretical and methodological problems inherent in researching sensitive topics (Brannen, 1988; Cannon, 1989; Lee, 1993; Liamputtong, 2007; Platzer & James, 1997; Renzetti & Lee, 1993; Robertson, 2000). What then, is the best way to approach a sensitive topic? Julia Brannen (1988:553) suggests that 'allowing the research topic to emerge gradually on its own terms is a theoretical as well as a methodological strategy'. Brannen (1988) adds that in researching sensitive topics it is important not to prejudge the research problem by labelling or defining the boundaries too closely. She feels that it is better to allow the participants to define the problem in their own terms.

Planning a sensitive research project

Collecting data in sensitive research can sometimes be a very difficult task and is often fraught with problems (Brannen, 1988; Lee, 1993; Renzetti & Lee, 1993). A number of methodological innovations have facilitated the collection of data on sensitive topics over the past 20 years; however, they have tended to be of the technical kind (Lee, 1993). These technological advances have focused on facilitating the asking of sensitive questions on surveys or methods to enhance the protection of confidentiality. In more recent years, the ethical, legal and political aspects of research have become more important (Lee, 1993). This has been coupled with a need to extend the research boundaries in an attempt to understand the lives of the people. Research on a sensitive topic that truly examines the experiences of people is more likely to be undertaken using qualitative methodologies (Liamputtong, 2007; see also Chapter 2 in this volume). This type of methodology is based on the interpretivist paradigm, which provides the researchers with a holistic approach to those involved in the research. It sees individuals in their social contexts and allows the research agenda to be shaped by both the researcher and the researched. It seeks to develop an understanding of the 'world view' of the research participants (Guba & Lincoln, 1985). Qualitative research is more suited to the study of sensitive topics as it does not assume prior knowledge of people's experiences (Lee, 1993). Instead it allows people to develop and express their own reality.

Many researchers of sensitive topics choose a qualitative design using the in-depth interview as their preferred method of data collection (Lee, 1993; Liamputtong, 2007). There is a range of issues that arise when qualitative interviewing is used by researchers investigating sensitive topics. One of the main issues raised is that these interviews are often stressful for both the researcher and the interviewee (Alty & Rodham, 1998; Burr, 1995; Campbell, 2002; Dunn, 1991; Gilbert, 2001b). In-depth interviews can be done on a one-off basis or they can involve a more longitudinal design. Some authors feel that sensitive research should be characterized by a one-off nature (Brannen, 1988); others feel that this is inappropriate and that we should first work at building rapport and a relationship with the potential participant through more than one interview (Oakley, 1981). Both approaches require the researcher to develop different kinds of relationships with the people they wish to involve in their research. There are a number of potential challenges associated with the types of relationships that researchers build with research participants. The intensity and duration of the relationship will vary with the different methodologies as well as the theoretical frameworks used to design the research.

Researchers choosing to conduct a one-off interview need to be aware that participants may be willing to disclose more to the researcher than they normally would due to the one-off nature of the encounter (Brannen, 1988). It has been found that building a relationship with a participant before beginning the research may also be problematic in that having an established relationship with a participant may impact on the types of information given to the researcher and may in fact be exploitative (Oakley, 1981) as participants may disclose more to a person whom they have established a relationship with. Sally Hutchinson, Margaret Wilson and Holly Skodol Wilson (1994) believe that people who cannot tolerate talking about a sensitive topic will not do so. However, as previously stated, if the researcher is able to build a relationship with the participant based on reciprocity and personal involvement then this may impact on their willingness to take part in the research and open a part of themselves that they ordinarily would keep closed. Some participants may not be aware of issues that taking part in research on a sensitive topic may evoke for them (Ramos, 1989). Research participants often do reveal highly personal aspects of their lives to researchers, which are beyond what people would normally disclose. While it is not possible to state whether a one-off encounter is better or worse than multiple-encounter research, it is important to note that the quality of the data collected may be dependent on the researcher's ability to develop an intimate and ongoing relationship with the participant.

One of the most important aspects of data collection in an in-depth interview on a sensitive topic is that the researcher is able to develop rapport with the participant (Johnson & Clarke, 2003; Lee, 1993; Liamputtong, 2007; Taylor & Bogdan, 1998). As stated by Victor Minichiello, Rosalie Aroni, Eric Timewell and Lois Alexander (2000:179):

> If we accept that in-depth interviewing necessitates establishing and maintaining good rapport with informants then it should also be recognised that such a process is never devoid of some form of emotional commitment from both sides of the fence.

Some researchers have reported experiencing feelings of guilt when the relationship comes to an end (Burr, 1995; Cannon, 1989). Others have spoken about the difficulties faced by researchers when the participants in their studies die (Beaver, Luker & Woods, 1999; Cannon, 1989, 1992; De Raeve, 1994).

Researchers need to be able to prepare themselves to physically and emotionally disengage at the end of the research. Minichiello and colleagues (2000:174) report that very few researchers prepare themselves to exit the relationship 'and even fewer report on the process when providing details of their project'. Some writers advocate for researchers to take into account the effects that exiting the research can have on both the researcher and the interviewee and the effect that this can have on the data (Lee-Treweek & Linkogle, 2000a; Ridge *et al.*, 1999). Ann Oakley (1981:41), a feminist methodologist, highlights that:

in most cases, the goal of finding out about people through interviewing is best achieved when the relationship of interviewer and interviewee is non-hierarchical and when the interviewer is prepared to invest his or her own personal identity in the relationship.

Part of this investment of personal identity in the research relationship involves researchers taking their and their participant's emotions into account in the collection and interpretation of the data. This emotion can take the form of verbal and non-verbal communication. For example pauses, silences and non-verbal emotional displays such as tears and embarrassment also need to be included in the data set and analysis. While there has been acknowledgement that there needs to be an emotional commitment made by researchers and participants, the impacts of making such a commitment have not been well documented.

Implications of researching a sensitive topic

Some researchers feel that undertaking research on a sensitive topic requires a thorough examination of the impacts that actually doing that research may have on both the researcher and the participant. For example, Kathleen Cowles (1988:164), in her research with a group of adult surviving relatives of murder victims carried out shortly after the murder, felt that:

Although aware of some of the potential problems related to the sensitivity of the topic and the vulnerability of the subjects, I was admittedly very naïve about the *actual* sensitivity and how the study activities would influence both the subjects and myself.

Researchers have often asked themselves questions about using vulnerable and disempowered people for their own research purposes (Liamputtong, 2007; Russell, 1999; Sque, 2000). The benefits of undertaking the research have to outweigh the risks of undertaking the research. This is a difficult problem as some of the issues surrounding sensitive research are not always apparent at the outset of the research. Researchers often cannot predict how they or the participants will be affected; they often do not know in advance what may come out of the research. Magi Sque (2000) raised this issue in her work with bereaved relatives of organ donors. She had a sense that she was dragging up painful memories for the sake of research. When researchers do gain entry into the private worlds of others they have the potential to invade, distort or destroy parts of the private world. If participants in sensitive research open themselves to this type of research they are also opening themselves to the possibility that they may be somehow changed by the process.

This is also true for the researchers. Researchers also open up some of themselves to the participants and in doing so render themselves vulnerable to change. Erving Goffman (1973:178) terms this a 'mortification of self', referring to a remaking of a person by an invasive exposure, as the embodiments of self are violated. In this 'mortification of self' he highlights that in order for people to have control over their lives they need to also have control over what is known about the private areas of their lives by others. By examining what often are painful experiences, sensitive research has the potential to invade or destroy this private world of both the participants and researchers. When researchers disclose parts of themselves to the participant to help build a relationship based on reciprocity and trust, they may in fact be rendering their own 'selves' as vulnerable.

Potential difficulties for the researcher

Raymond Lee (1993) in his book *Doing Research on Sensitive Topics* presents many of the threats and difficulties that may be faced by both the participants and the researchers. In the introduction he states that: 'Sensitive research often also has potential effects on the personal life, and sometimes on the personal security, of the researcher' (Lee, 1993:1). In this statement he alerts researchers that undertaking sensitive research can impact on aspects of their personal lives. Warnings like these are not new. Since the early 1970s researchers have been thinking and writing about the potential effects that social research can have on the researcher (Kellehear, 1989; Liamputtong, 2007; Perry, 1989; Sieber & Stanley, 1988; Wax, 1971). While these writings have focused on social research in general, Lee (1993) was the first author to concentrate specifically on the issues for researchers of sensitive research topics. In presenting the issues for these researchers, Raymond Lee (1993:16) highlights that:

researchers need to find ways of dealing with the problems and issues raised by research on sensitive topics. The threats which the research poses to research participants, to the researcher and to others need to minimized, managed or mitigated.

Researchers have become particularly adept at assessing and mitigating any threats or harms to the participants that may be inherent in the research. However, doing the same for the researchers is yet to be fully developed and accepted by the research community.

Although research on sensitive topics may evoke some kinds of emotional distress in some people it can also have some positive effects. Sally Hutchinson, Margaret Wilson and Holly Wilson (1994) outline some of the benefits of participating in research interviews including catharsis, sense of purpose, helping others, empowerment, healing, having a voice, and being heard. Other researchers have also mentioned that their participants felt relief and a sense of catharsis from the sharing of their stories (Brannen, 1988, 1993; Cowles, 1988; Lee & Renzetti, 1993; Owens, 1996; Platzer & James, 1997; Sque, 2000). Many participants do find research both enjoyable and personally rewarding (Cook & Bosley, 1995; Hutchinson *et al.*, 1994; Kondora, 1993; Liamputtong, 2007; Liamputtong Rice, 2000). Claire Draucker (1999:164) states that her participants felt that 'their participation was beneficial to them, usually because it gave them an opportunity to share their thoughts and feelings and possibly help other victims of violence'. So, while some participants may also take part in research for altruistic reasons, the participants themselves may gain from their participation. It has been stated that research is always an intervention and that people can be changed in the process of participating in research. Michael Quinn Patton (1990:353) expresses his ideas:

Interviews are interventions. They affect people. A good interview lays open thoughts, feelings, knowledge and experience not only to the interviewer but also to the interviewee. A process of being taken through a directed, reflective process affects the person being interviewed and leaves them knowing things about themselves that they didn't know – or at least were not aware of – before the interview. Two hours or more of thoughtfully reflecting on an experience, a program or one's life can be change inducing. Yet the purpose of a research interview is first and foremost to gather data, not change people.

Many researchers grapple with this idea of research as an intervention. All research is essentially an intervention; all research has the ability to offer people different perspectives on their lives. Although researchers need to remember that the ultimate goal of research is to gather data, they cannot dismiss the idea that in gathering that data they may be providing the participants with a chance to assess certain aspects of their lives.

Summary

This book comprises seven chapters. In this chapter we have discussed the different definitions of sensitive research and examined some of the topics that may be considered sensitive. An outline of the issues to consider when planning a research project on a sensitive issue has been provided. We have explored some of the historical developments in sensitive research and discussed their relevance for public health research.

In Chapter 2 we outline the theoretical and practical issues relative to choosing a methodology. We will examine the methods literature relevant to the qualitative/quantitative debate and discuss the decision to adopt a qualitative methodology for the study of researchers' experiences of undertaking sensitive research.

Chapter 3 presents the 'story' of conducting sensitive qualitative research as told by researchers working in the field of sensitive health research. In this chapter we provide an overview of the conduct and process of undertaking qualitative research on a sensitive topic and raise some important points for researchers to consider throughout the research process. These include issues relating to rapport development, use of researcher self-disclosure, listening to untold stories, feelings of guilt and vulnerability, leaving the research relationship and researcher exhaustion.

Qualitative health researchers immerse themselves in the settings that they are studying, which results in personal interaction with research participants. As a result of this immersion, the boundaries between the researcher and the group of people under study can easily become 'blurred'. In Chapter 4 we focus particularly on the boundary issues inherent in sensitive research including boundaries between researcher/friend, researcher and counsellor/therapist and self/other. We conclude this chapter with a discussion of the implications of poor boundary management for researchers and strategies for ensuring effective boundary management.

There is a growing awareness that undertaking qualitative research on sensitive topics is an embodied experience and that researchers may be emotionally affected by the work that they do. In Chapter 5 we examine a number of different conceptualizations of emotions and explore their relevance for research work on sensitive topics. The sociological literature pertinent to emotion work is explored. We describe the theories of emotion work and how they might be applied to the experience of undertaking sensitive research. The chapter concludes with discussion of the implications for researchers undertaking emotion work and offers some suggestions for researcher self-care.

While ethics committees and research supervisors are well versed in assessing risks to potential participants in sensitive research, the risks for the actual researchers and other members of the research team are often not considered. In Chapter 6 we provide an overview of risk theory, examine risks in sensitive research and offer some discussion regarding roles and responsibilities of risk assessment and management. The ethical issues, including confidentiality, anonymity and reviews of the role of ethics committees in assessing potential harm to researchers, are also discussed. Based on evidence from the field this chapter argues that there is currently insufficient recognition of the need for protection of researchers and other members of the research team involved in qualitative research on sensitive topics.

In Chapter 7 we outline the implications for researchers of our findings and provide a number of recommendations for practice and policy. These recommendations are tailored for specific groups in the research process, including researchers, transcribers, and research supervisors, universities, granting bodies, research centres and ethics committees. Adoption of these recommendations will ensure that qualitative research on sensitive topics can continue to be conducted without adversely affecting those who are involved in it.

Tutorial activities

(a) Earlier in this chapter we provided a number of different definitions of what constitutes 'sensitive research'. Review these definitions and then brainstorm to produce a list of at least ten topics that could be considered sensitive. Identify why each topic is sensitive and classify as personal, taboo or emotional.

(b) Now select three of the topics from the list you generated in (a) above. Conduct a search of a literature database or of hard copy journals at your institution library and try to find at least one qualitative research paper describing research on each topic. Which topics were easy to find information on? Which topics were difficult? Do the authors in any of the papers discuss challenges they faced in conducting qualitative research on this topic?

SUGGESTED READING

Daly, J., Kellehear, A. & Gliksman, M. (1997). *The Public Health Researcher*. Melbourne: Oxford University Press.

Johnson, B. & Clarke, J. (2003). Collecting sensitive data: the impact on the researchers. *Qualitative Health Research*, **13**(3), 421–434.

Lee, R.M. (1993). *Doing Research on Sensitive Topics*. London: Sage Publications.

Liamputtong, P. (2007). *Researching the Vulnerable: A Guide to Sensitive Research Methods*. London: Sage Publications.

Renzetti, C. & Lee, R.M. (eds.) (1993). *Researching Sensitive Topics*. Newbury Park: Sage Publications.

Sieber, J.E. & Stanley, B. (1988). Ethical and professional dimensions of socially sensitive research. *American Psychologist*, **43**, 49–55.

2

Doing sensitive research: methodological, theoretical, ethical and moral perspectives

Knowledge is subjective, constructed and based on the shared signs and symbols that are recognized by members of a culture. Multiple realities are presumed, with different people experiencing these differently.

(Grbich, 2007:8)

In any piece of research, it is typical that we should include the theoretical framework that we base our research on. This is the main focus of this chapter. In this chapter, we will first discuss the theoretical issues relative to choosing a methodology. We will examine the methods literature relevant to the qualitative/quantitative debate and discuss the decision to adopt a qualitative methodology for the study of researchers' experiences of undertaking sensitive research. We will also discuss the issues of intrusion, ethical, moral and legal issues in the second part of this chapter.

Debates in the philosophy of science

In designing this study, it was important for us to examine a number of ontological and epistemological questions that underlie how research is conducted. The ontological question revolves around a discussion of whether or not there is a single objective reality (Denzin & Lincoln, 2005a). The epistemological question relates to the nature of knowledge and how knowledge can be obtained (Guba & Lincoln, 1994). In many of the classic texts, there is an argument about whether or not social science research can be objective (see Daly, 2007; Denzin & Lincoln, 2005a; Grbich, 2007; Willis, 2007). Max Weber (1949) maintains that social science could be value free. However, other philosophers such as Jürgen Habermas strongly question Weber's thesis, challenging the illusion of objectivist research (Habermas, 1971, 1988). Habermas asserts that the search for the 'truth' is in fact futile because there is no such thing as 'truth'. Instead he reminds us that we, as researchers, should not be concerned about searching for truth as all knowledge is socially constructed and the creation of such knowledge needs both the researcher and the research participant to engage with each other. If one assumes the ontological notion of objective reality then the knower (that is, the researcher/scientist) must assume the position of objective detachment that is free from all bias. In adopting this standpoint, objectivist researchers believe that reality can be accurately captured (Grbich, 2007). In contrast to this position, if a researcher rejected the notion of objectivity, then it is not necessary to conduct research in a detached and dispassionate way. In his rejection of objectivist research, Anthony Giddens (1993) contends that researchers always influence what they research. In order to understand the experiences and realities of another, the researcher needs to acknowledge their own subjectivities (for example, values, beliefs and emotions) and how they are involved in the research process.

Egon Guba and Yvonna Lincoln (1994) propose that within the social sciences, there are four major epistemological theories that are used to explain the nature of knowledge: positivism, postpositivism, critical theory and constructivism. All of these traditions offer the researcher a different understanding of what reality is and how we can come to know that reality (Broom & Willis, 2007; Willis, 2007).

Positivism holds the ontological belief of 'naïve realism' that there is an objective reality that can be accessed (Guba & Lincoln, 1994). Therefore, the positivistic goal of scientific inquiry is to explain, predict or control that reality. One of the central ideas of positivist methodologies is the generation and testing of hypotheses through scientific means. Carol Grbich (2007:4) says this clearly:

Positivism views truth as absolute and values the original and unique aspects of scientific research such as realistic descriptions, truthful depiction, studies which have clear aims, objectives and properly measured outcomes, a focus on neutrality, objectivity (knowledge of reality gained by a neutral and distant researcher utilising reason, logic and a range of carefully pre-tested research tools) and theory testing that can distinguish between facts and values.

As such, positivistic research does not allow for the researcher's personal point of view or emotions to enter into the research process (Guba & Lincoln, 2005). This type of involvement and the presence of emotion in research are seen as a 'taboo'. Marjorie DeVault (1997:220) criticizes this type of research, examining the positivistic concerns that personal and emotional involvement in research may somehow impede these claims to 'truth'. Traditional research methodologies and designs are heavily influenced by scientific positivism and the patriarchal academic structures that accompany it, as it is seen 'the crowning achievement of Western civilization' (Denzin & Lincoln, 2005a:8).

There is an ideology built up that encourages researchers to be aware of personal and emotional involvement and to put in place a number of strategies to prevent it from happening. In adopting this tradition, it is paramount that the scientist (researcher) must be objective and free from bias that may interfere with gathering the data (Guba & Lincoln, 2005). The researcher's human qualities should not enter into the scientific research process. In their practice, positivism takes the stance that 'truth can transcend opinion and personal bias' and as such, a qualitative approach, which is based on a constructivist paradigm (see below), is seen as 'an assault' on the positivist approach (Denzin & Lincoln, 2005a:8).

The second tradition is postpositivism (sometime referred to as realism) and is underpinned by some of the positivistic characteristics that we discussed above with some slight deviations. Postpositivists believe that there is an objective reality that can be captured but it is impossible to capture it in a pure, unbiased form, hence, most adhere to 'critical realism' (see Guba & Lincoln, 1994). Postpositivism, as Grbich (2007:6) contends, 'asserts that structures creating the world cannot always be directly observed (as in positivism), and when and if they are observable their genesis is not always clear; thus we also need our creative minds to clarify their existence and then to identify explanatory mechanisms'. And research in a realist approach emphasizes 'the identification of the linking of different realisms'. Within this framework, it is important for researchers to identify and remove all sources of bias in their search for the 'truth'.

In their recent piece, Egon Guba and Yvonna Lincoln (2005:184) point to the similarities between positivism and postpositivism, which include: its 'reliance on naïve realism, dualistic epistemologies, verificational approach to inquiry, emphasis on reliability, validity, prediction, control, and a building block approach to knowledge'. These two paradigms, they suggest, have their limitations in addressing 'issues surrounding voice, empowerment, and praxis' adequately.

The ontology of critical theorists is 'historical realism' and most believe that there is no one objective reality but that reality is interpreted through social, political, cultural, economic, ethnic and gender values (Guba & Lincoln, 1994). The goal of research in this tradition is to understand how the values of both the researcher and the participants determine how they see the world. Often, critical theorists emphasize the influence of power relationships between members of society and are oriented toward emancipation and empowerment of the participants and hope to bring about social transformation toward more justice and equity in the world (Guba & Lincoln, 2005; Willis, 2007). For critical theorists, it is not enough for researchers just to do research with powerless people, but the research process and results must also be utilized in a way that will help the powerless to deal with or eradicate problems in their everyday lives. Jerry Willis (2007:85) puts this clearly:

Critical theory's idealized version of what research should be is based on the concept that the research process is interwoven with practice in such a way that it helps those who are oppressed to free themselves from the oppression.

Nevertheless, there are different critical theorist traditions (see Guba & Lincoln, 1994). Critical theorists who take a more postpositivist orientation believe that the identity of the 'knower' is important because the beliefs, values and experiences of that person shape how the research is conceptualized, how data is collected and how the research findings are interpreted. Critical postpostivist researchers acknowledge that it is not possible to filter out these factors and so they must be open in articulating how their own experiences shape the findings of the research. In their recent piece, Egon Guba and Yvonna Lincoln (2005:204) explain this clearly:

Rather than locating foundational truth and knowledge in some external reality 'out there', such critical theorists tend to locate the foundations of truth in specific, historical, economic, racial, and social infrastructures of oppression, injustice, and marginalization.

Constructivists take the ideas of the critical theorists one step further and argue that 'reality' is socially constructed, shaped by social factors such as age, gender, race, class and culture (Grbich, 2007). Its ontology is 'relativist' (Guba & Lincoln, 1994). Constructivist researchers explicitly reject the ideal of a single truth and instead believe that there are multiple truths that are individually constructed (see for example Guba & Lincoln, 1994, 2005; Grbich, 2007; Willis, 2007). One of the central beliefs of researchers working in this paradigm is their belief that research is a very subjective process due to the active involvement of the researcher in the construction and conduct of the research (Grbich, 2007). Research situated within this standpoint, as Carol Grbich (2007:8) points out, focuses on 'exploration of the way people interpret and make sense of their experiences in the worlds in which they live, and how the contexts of events and situations and the placement of these within wider social environments have impacted on constructed understanding'.

Many qualitative, constructionist researchers reject the use of quantitative, positivist assumptions and methods (Denzin & Lincoln, 2005a). Positivist methods, for some researchers, are just one way of 'telling stories about societies or social worlds'. These methods may not be better or worse than any other methods, but they 'tell different kind of stories'. Others will have little or no tolerance to this view. They believe that the criteria used in positivist science are 'irrelevant to their work' and argue that 'such criteria reproduce only a certain kind of science, a science that silences too many voices'.

Positivism and postpositivism dominate quantitative social science research whereas qualitative research is influenced by critical theory and interpretivism

(Willis, 2007). In order to undertake the research on which this book is based, we have adopted a constructivist stance acknowledging the very subjective nature of the research and the multiple realities of those involved in the research. And as such, this necessitated the use of qualitative methodology.

Qualitative methodology

The province of qualitative research . . . is the world of lived experience, for this is where individual belief and action intersect with culture. (Denzin & Lincoln, 2005a:8)

Qualitative methodologies are particularly suited to constructivist researchers who are interested in researching experiences from the standpoint of those who are living them (Charmaz, 2000). A research design should reflect the research aim, questions and the epistemological understandings that are appropriate to the study (Grbich, 1999; Liamputtong & Ezzy, 2005). We do not wish to debate the merits of qualitative over quantitative methods in any great detail as this is ongoing in the literature (Denzin & Lincoln, 2000; Grbich, 1999). However, it is important to understand that qualitative research is ontologically and epistemologically grounded in the interpretive paradigm (Denzin & Lincoln, 2005b). In this paradigm, researchers are neither engaged in a search for 'truth', nor are they focused on discovering one 'reality'.

Researchers grounded in this paradigm advocate for the acknowledgement of multiple truths and multiple realities (Denzin & Lincoln, 2005b; Daly, 2007). In order to understand this, Weber's concept of *vertstehen* can be applied (Weber, 1949). This concept was initially formulated by Max Weber and further developed by later theorists. It is characterized by a process of subjective interpretation on the part of the researcher, which includes a degree of sympathetic understanding between the researcher and the participants in the study, whereby the researcher comes to share, in part, the situated meanings and experiences of those under study. Applying this concept makes it possible to bridge the dualisms of researcher and researched by developing the researcher's own experiences and emotions in order to access the meanings of the situation and the experiences of the participants.

Qualitative research based in the interpretive paradigm is exploratory in nature, thus enabling researchers to gain information about areas in which little is known (Liamputtong & Ezzy, 2005). A qualitative approach was chosen for our study as we aimed to understand the experience of undertaking qualitative research on sensitive topics from the researcher's perspective. As highlighted by Victor Minichiello and colleagues (2000:11): 'the focus of qualitative research is not to reveal causal relationships, but rather to discover the nature of phenomena as humanly experienced'. We as qualitative researchers, as Denzin and Lincoln (2005a:10) put it: 'stress the socially constructed nature of reality, the intimate relationship between the researcher and what is studied, and the situational constraints that shape inquiry'. We 'seek answers to questions that stress how social experience is created and given meaning'. We contend that taking a constructivist approach to the research on which this book is based has enabled us to document the human experience of doing sensitive research from the perspective of the researcher.

Feminist frameworks

There are many parallels in the values that underpin constructivist and feminist approaches to research. The theoretical frameworks of feminist interpretive research and constructivism differ from the positivist nature of conventional scientific research, with both frameworks acknowledging that knowledge is socially constructed, shaped by social factors such as age, gender, race, class and culture (Hesse-Biber & Leavy, 2005; Liamputtong, 2007; Olesen, 2005). Traditionally, the construction of knowledge was based on principles like objectivity and generalizability, the foundations of the scientific method. This method has been heavily criticized by feminist researchers due to its androcentric and hierarchical nature (Harding, 1987; Oakley, 1981; Smith, 1987). The goal of interpretive research is 'to make the world of problematic lived experience of ordinary people directly available to the reader' (Denzin, 1989:7). Initially derived from phenomenology (Husserl, 1970; Van Maanen, 1990a) and later embraced by feminist researchers, the study of lived experience aims to both describe and interpret experiences of everyday life.

Feminist researchers use the same methods that many other researchers do; however, the ways in which the methods are used differs from those of more 'androcentric researchers' (Mies, 1983:118). Qualitative research based in the interpretive paradigm is an excellent method for feminist researchers to use to increase their understanding of how people view their experiences. In order to gain an understanding of people's experience, many feminist researchers advocate for qualitative methods and more particularly in-depth interviews and oral history, as a method of data gathering (Campbell & Wasco, 2000; Liamputtong, 2007; Reinharz, 1992). It has been argued that these principles of feminist research are particularly relevant when undertaking research on sensitive topics (Bergen, 1993; Klein, 1983; Renzetti & Lee, 1993).

Many feminist researchers have been critical of the methodological and epistemological underpinnings of research over the past few decades (Klein, 1983; Oakley, 1981; Ribbens & Edwards, 1998; Stanley & Wise, 1990, 1993). Although we have seen some contemporary feminist researchers promote both positivist and constructivist methods in recent years (Campbell, 2002; Campbell & Salem, 1999; Campbell & Wasco, 2000), many feminist researchers reject the positivistic ideal that the researcher should, or even can, remain an objective observer. Researchers advocating for research based on feminist principles encourage active involvement of both the researcher and the participant in the research (Liamputtong, 2007). This involves building and facilitating a reciprocal relationship between the researcher and the participant using a number of different strategies. Research relationships based on feminist principles advocate for reciprocity and collaboration including answering questions based on personal experiences, some level of self-disclosure and the formation of friendships with research participants (Oakley, 1981).

In contrast to this position, Cotterill (1992) questions the effectiveness of the reciprocal process, arguing that some distance between researcher and participant is preferable. She terms this relationship the 'friendly stranger', contending that the researcher, unlike a friend, 'does not exercise social control over respondents because the relationship exists for the purpose of research and is terminated when the research is complete' (Cotterill, 1992:596).

Researchers working from within a feminist interpretive perspective are also openly encouraged to provide an honest accountability of the researcher's contribution to and effect on any research project (Harding, 1991; Stanley & Wise, 1993). Liz Stanley and Sue Wise (1991:266) have observed that in many research texts the 'research process appears a very orderly and coherent process', often not providing a true reflection of how the researcher was involved in the process. They have termed research lacking personal state-ments and feeling 'hygenic research', positing that this research is research that is described rather than experienced. For researchers to gain access to private and often intimate parts of people's lives, it is important that they give something of themselves to the participants (Liamputtong, 2007). Jane Ribbens and Rosalind Edwards (1998:203) ask the question, 'are we looking for openness from our research participants that we are not willing to show about ourselves?' This openness and reflexivity is paramount in qualitative research based on constructivist and feminist research principles.

Embodied research

Embodiment theory is in contrast to much of the thinking in Western thought of the mind/body split more commonly referred to as Cartesian dualism (Turner, 1992). Cartesian dualism presupposes that the person is made of two completely separate parts, one the mind and the other the body. One of the main assertions of embodiment is that to be human means that all parts of the body are integral and one part cannot be separated from the other. Much of the research in health and social science has accepted the Cartesian legacy of separation of mind and body. Thus, the body became the subject of the 'natural' sciences, leaving the mind for the humanities (Lupton, 1995; Turner, 1992). Embodiment can be defined in a way that reflects the phenomenological philosophy of Merleau-Ponty (1962) relating to how we live in and experience the world through our bodies, especially through things such as perception, emotion and language (Merleau-Ponty, 1962). The body is the means by which we, as humans, come to know and experience the world (Merleau-Ponty, 1962). The importance of the body in social interaction has been well documented (Goffman, 1959). This embodiment is the avenue for much of Merleau-Ponty's ontology and epistemology focusing on how existence is known through the body. He describes how subject and object are related to one another in the world with the body having two aspects; the sentient (phenomenal) and the sensible (objective). An example of this could be seen in human abilities such as being able to touch and be touched both physically and emotionally by another person. Sue Cataldi (1993:129) puts it this way: 'To say that we have been 'touched' or that an situation was 'touching' is synonymous with saying that we have been emotionally affected'.

Researchers working in health research do not often communicate the embodied aspects of the research experience. Embodied existence takes place within the contextual world that each person is born into and lives in. This world is essentially shaped by culture, society, history and personal relation-ships and it must be interpreted to be understood. As embodied beings, we come to know the world through shared understandings, and in the process make our experience of the world a social and intersubjective one. All aspects of research require the researcher to feel, to experience. As researchers, we are 'embodied', situated and subjective in the analysis.

Undertaking an inquiry into a sensitive issue (e.g. cancer, domestic vio-lence, rape, abortion, miscarriage, addiction, living with HIV/AIDS and disability) cannot be readily studied using structured type questionnaires or surveys as these often rely on themes that have been predetermined. As Kerry Daly (2007) and Pranee Liamputtong (2007) have pointed out, predeter-mined responses cannot easily capture the experience of sensitive issues. Getting people to disclose about aspects of their private lives has and con-tinues to challenge many social scientists. Studying sensitive topics or emotive topics requires a research method that enables the researcher to respond in a sensitive way to the concerns of the participant. Researchers need to be able to listen, be empathetic and to allow the person to tell their story. We are facilitators of that process for people. Researchers on sensitive topics need time and to build a certain level of trust and rapport before a person will disclose intimate or sensitive information.

Subjectivity of qualitative research on sensitive topics

Undertaking all qualitative research is a subjective experience regardless of which framework is adopted. Researchers cannot hide behind the mask of objectivity and pretend that they are not intimately involved in the research that they do. The subjective nature of qualitative research is particularly evident to researchers studying sensitive topics (Liamputtong, 2007). We, like Stanley and Wise (1993:113), '. . . reject the idea of 'the researcher' as a god-like creature who is able to leave behind subjective involvements' while conducting research. As previously stated, these researchers must develop special relationships with participants in order to document their experiences. When undertaking qualitative research, the researchers are the data collection instrument; they interact with participants in order to collect data for their studies. Doing this type of research requires human interaction and qualitative researchers cannot remain faceless interviewers, they must invest part of themselves in order to collect the data (Fontana & Frey, 1994). In doing so, qualitative researchers, and more particularly qualitative researchers researching sensitive topics, need to be aware of their subjectivity. Carolyn Ellis (1991) calls for researchers not to be embarrassed about their subjectivity, alerting us to the fact that our personal stories remind people that emotions are not just the exclusive property of the people we research.

One of the problems with researchers being openly subjective in their research is that this type of openness is undervalued and regarded by some as contaminating to the data. It has been highlighted that many researchers publish what have been termed 'objective' research reports and then later publish additional papers that purport to 'tell it like it is' (Stanley & Wise, 1993:60). The problem with this is that it only allows researchers access to the more objectively written papers, thus adding to the devaluation of subjectivity in research. Researchers do, for many reasons, remove or fail to report the personal in their research writings and it is rare to find a frank discussion of what the process of doing the research was like. Liz Stanley and Sue Wise (1991:266) say it clearly:

The personal tends to be carefully removed from public statements; these are full of rational argument and careful discussion of academic points of dispute and are frequently empty of any feeling of what the research process was actually like.

Much research literature concentrates on its discussions about ethics, informed consent, access and dealing with gatekeepers. Although all of these are very important issues in any research, so are the discussions that give some insight into the personal issues that the research may have raised for the researcher or others involved (Fonow & Cook, 1991; Stanley & Wise, 1991). If researchers continually remove reference to the realities of the research process from their writings, the difficulties associated with doing research, particularly on sensitive topics, are likely to remain hidden. Research is a subjective experience, which requires researchers to be aware of their own role in the production of knowledge; parallel to this is the need for reflexivity (Hughes, 1998; May, 1998).

Reflexivity

Reflexivity is central to both constructivist and feminist research (Allen & Walker, 1992; Liamputtong, 2007; Stanko, 1997) and being reflexive in research demands that the researcher engage on a number of different levels with the research. Reflexive researchers need to have an awareness of their own responses, beliefs and prejudices (Hertz, 1997; Morley, 1996; Ribbens & Edwards, 1998). It is one of the central tenets of research based on feminist principles (Campbell & Wasco, 2000; Darlington & Scott, 2002; DeVault, 1997; Hertz, 1997; Jansen & Davis, 1998; Ribbens & Edwards, 1998; Stanley & Wise, 1991). Being reflexive in research requires the researcher to document the research process and locate themselves in that process because, 'the subjectivity of the researcher herself is part of the research production' (Harrison & Lyon, 1993:105). Many feminist researchers advocate for reflexivity throughout the whole research as it enables us, as sensitive researchers, to learn from the process. As Rosanna Hertz (1997:viii) states, 'to be reflexive is to have an ongoing conversation about the experience while simultaneously living in the moment'.

As feminist research comes from a tradition that openly supports both self-examination and sharing, researchers should undertake to ensure that their research reflects these goals (Fonow & Cook, 1991; Stanley & Wise, 1991). Reflexivity requires the researcher to be openly aware of the ways in which self affects both the research process and the outcomes of the research (Gergen & Gergen, 1991; Liamputtong & Ezzy, 2005). In reporting the findings of research, it is important that there is an awareness of the ways in which the researcher's self affects both the processes and outcomes. Egon Guba and Yvonna Lincoln (2005:210) say that 'reflexivity forces us to come to terms not only with our choice of research problem and with those with whom we engage in the research process, but with our selves and with the multiple identities that represent the fluid self in the research setting'. Shulamit Reinharz (1997:3) too argues that we, as researchers, 'bring the self to the field . . . [we also] create the self in the field'. We too believe this is the essence of sensitive researchers when we work with marginalized and vulnerable people in our research endeavours.

Recently, we have seen this type of report writing emerging in the social science areas. Often, these are referred to as autoethnographical texts (Ellis, 2004; Ellis & Bochner, 2000; Ellis & Bochner, 1996; Jones, 2005; Richardson, 1994; Richardson & Lockeridge, 2004; Richardson & St Pierre, 2005). Some feminist writers have put their 'self' in their writing and they are not ashamed to do so either (Ellis, 1995; Jones, 2005; Letherby, 2000; Richardson, 1997; Ronai, 1995, 1996; Ronai & Ellis, 2001).

Sensitive research: political, ethical and moral perspectives

In researching sensitive topics, there are several issues that sensitive researchers must consider before embarking on their research enterprises.

Issue of intrusion

One of the main ethical issues is the issue of intrusion. Any person undertaking sensitive research will be asked by an ethics committee whether or not the research could be carried out another way other than talking with people. Could an existing database be adopted for researching sensitive topics?

When people talk about doing qualitative research, most immediately think about talking with people either individually or in groups, or participating in other people activities. However, as Allan Kellehear (1993a) argues, some research may not necessitate talking with people or participating in their routines when an answer to the research question may be found in existing literature and research. There are also some data that it may not be feasible to collect because of political sensitivity or simply because the informants no longer exist for researchers to interview. Furthermore, if the research questions deal with delicate situations or groups of people, such as people with HIV/AIDS or indigenous people, should the researcher intrude into these people's private lives when there is existing information that has not yet been examined (Kellehear, 1997)? Unobtrusive methods can offer answers to these situations.

Even when people tell you what they believe or do in the interview situation, do they tell you the truth? They may not do so because of some personal, social, cultural or political situations. Because of the limitations in talking to people, Allan Kellehear (1993a:48) argues that unobtrusive methods 'help restore meaning and context to confessions of belief, attitude and knowledge'. This is particularly so when unobtrusive methods are used with other qualitative methods.

If there is no other way to obtain original data other than intruding in to the life of vulnerable groups, sensitive researchers must think carefully what methodological steps will be taken to 'lessen the intrusion' (Kellehear, 1997). For example, rather than doing an in-depth or a long interview, which requires the participants to spend a long period of time for the research purpose and most often is very intrusive, the use of observations, shortened interview schedules, participant observation and participatory action research methods may be adopted (Kellehear, 1997). Kellehear (1993b) even suggests that the employment of questionnaires instead of long interviews may work very well in sensitive research. In his earlier research with dying people,

Kellehear (1990) employed a survey method because of the issue of intrusion that researchers tend to impose on vulnerable people. In his study, cancer patients 'had trouble holding their concentration or controlling their pain, vomiting or nausea' and 'others found our discussions emotionally draining' (Kellehear, 1993b:131). In this instance, it would be extremely unethical for sensitive researchers to impose on the participants a long and in-depth interviewing method, and as such an imaginatively developed survey might be the answer. Allan Kellehear (1993b:137) puts this clearly:

Health research is commonly conducted with and by people who enjoy reasonable physical health. However, research with the very old, the chronically ill and the acutely ill is increasing . . . But the desire by many researchers for time-consuming, unstructured conversations may not sit well or be easily accommodated by these populations of sick people. Given that constraint, and put in that context, the survey may well do with being reconsidered occasionally.

Although we agree with the point Kellehear has suggested, in our research we felt that the unobtrusive methods would not allow us to fully understand the lived experiences of researchers who have engaged in sensitive research. At the time this research was being undertaken, there were hardly any publications dedicated to doing sensitive research. However, several publications have since emerged in journals and books. The observation method, including direct and participant observations, was not feasible for us to carry out due to time constraints. Most researchers we interviewed in this research were busy academic and research staff. Hence, an in-depth interviewing method was our primary data collection method in this study.

Ethical issues

Ethics is a set of moral principles that aims to prevent researchers from harming those they research. Ethics and politics are important in the study of sensitive topics as politics is about the strategies that we use to gain a position of power in the research. Researchers undertaking research on sensitive topics need to be acutely aware of their ethical responsibilities (Lee, 1993; Liamputtong, 2007). The four ethical principles of respect for autonomy (informed consent), non-maleficence (do no harm), beneficence (benefits of the research outweigh the risks) and justice (research strategies are fair and just) provide the framework for ensuring that the rights of research participants are upheld (Beauchamp & Childress, 1994).

These basic ethical principles should form the basis of all research. However, when undertaking sensitive research, consideration of these guidelines alone may not be sufficient to undertake a full assessment of the risks of the research. This framework for ethical assessment does not specifically require researchers to reflect on the ethical issues that may arise in the research related to the researcher as well as to the participant. Researchers have raised the issue of the 'emergent nature' and unpredictability of qualitative research. This further complicates the ethics process as researchers may have difficulty in undertaking a full assessment of the ethical issues before the research actually begins (Robertson, 2000). The ethical issues inherent in undertaking sensitive research will be discussed in more detail in Chapter 6.

Moral perspective and sensitive research

Similar to the issue of intrusion, there are some debates about moral issues regarding sensitive research. If we claim to be sensitive researchers, should we carry out research with some people who are vulnerable and marginalized, such as homeless people, frail elderly, terminally ill persons, people suffering mental illness, or those who experience extreme loss and grief, when these people are already vulnerable in so many ways? In her attempt to do research on social isolation with older people in Sydney, Australia, Cherry Russell (1999:404) and her co-researchers asked themselves, for example 'should we be 'mining the minds' of these disempowered people for our own research purposes?'. In order to be responsive to their participants, they modified many aspects of their research, but throughout the research process they encountered 'a sense of unease about the ethicality (or even morality) of some aspects of their research'.

Nevertheless, some researchers have shown that this is not always the case (see Stanley, Stanley, Lautin et al., 1981; Usher & Holmes, 1997). In fact, as Kim Usher and Colin Holmes (1997) contend, people with mental illness may wish to take part in a research project despite the paternalistic view of their caregivers, advocates, guardians or family members. In their research with homeless people, Tom Beauchamp and colleagues (2002:560) argue similarly that it is not immoral or exploitative to include homeless people in research if it is carried out ethically. Jan Morse (2000) goes a step further in arguing for doing research with some extremely vulnerable people. Morse (2000:545) puts it bluntly that:

It is immoral not to conduct research with the critically ill or dying; they are the most disenfranchised members of our society and most in need of understanding. Qualitative research can provide insights into their experiences, their discomforts, and their needs and show how care can be improved and their needs met.

Morse argues that conducting research with extremely vulnerable people 'is good in the moral sense'. We would also argue that it is morally important to gain knowledge about people with terminal illnesses if we aim to achieve a service provision of a high quality that meets their needs (see Beaver et al., 1999).

Ethics of care and sensitive research

Carol Gilligan (1977, 1982) proposes an ethic of care that emphasizes care, compassion and relationships (see also Held, 1993; Israel & Hay, 2006;

Noddings, 2003). An ethic of care demands that 'the search for just outcomes to ethical problems takes account of care, compassion, and our interpersonal relationships, and ties to families and groups' (Israel & Hay, 2006:22). This ethics of care has marked ramifications for moral and ethical issues in undertaking sensitive research. Following Gilligan's ethics of care, we propose several ethics of care in undertaking sensitive research here.

Morally and ethically responsible researchers need to take 'the personal, interpersonal, community, and political ramifications of research' (Paradis, 2000:854) on their research participants into consideration when carrying out sensitive research. In a study involving homeless women, for example, Emily Paradis (2000:854) contends that researchers must recognize that 'homeless women are very vulnerable to harm as individuals, and as a community because of the extreme victimization, stigmatization and marginalization they endure'. The moral challenge for sensitive researchers is then to develop their inquiries in ways that do not make the individual participants suffer further.

Many sensitive researchers strongly believe that the benefits of undertaking the research need to be weighed against the risks or other inconveniences of being involved in the research (Cutcliffe & Ramcharan, 2002; Hall & Kuilg, 2004; Israel & Hay, 2006; Liamputtong, 2007). Although risks and harm applies to all research, it is more pertinent in sensitive research as this may make people more vulnerable. Maggie O'Neill (1996), Priscilla Pyett (2001) and Deborah Warr (2004) for example, suggest that undertaking research with women working on the street has moral ramifications for the women themselves. The times the women have to spend in our research can have a negative impact on their contacts with their clients.

The moral issue of questions that researchers ask in their study with vulnerable people has been raised by many sensitive researchers (Liamputtong, 2007). As a moral and sensitive researcher, we should not ask questions that may contribute to the stigmatization of our research participants. In research with homeless women that she was involved with, Emily Paradis (2000) makes a strong case advocating for asking research questions that would reflect better on the marginalized lives of these women. This essentially necessitates the use of qualitative research questions, rather than hypothesis testing in positivist science.

The issue of self-disclosure of the research participants has been raised by sensitive researchers (Etherington, 1996; France, Bendelow & Williams, 2000; Liamputtong, 2007; Melrose, 2002). Unanticipated disclosure may occur in research with vulnerable people. Through the process of talking in depth, people might disclose more about their lived experiences than they thought they would do (Henslin, 2001; Lupton, 1998; Meadows, Lagendyk, Thurston et al., 2003; Seymour, Bellamy, Gott et al., 2002). Kerry Daly (1992) also suggests that the inherent power imbalance between researchers and research participants may result in disclosure, as some participants may feel obligated to respond to questions they would not otherwise answer. Although sometimes it is beyond our control, researchers should actively encourage their participants not to talk about others in the interview by reminding them of privacy issues or asking the participants to withdraw segments of data from the record so that the privacy of other people may not be breached. This type of situation can be problematic for both the researcher and the participants. As sensitive researchers, we must develop our own strategies for handling these types of difficulties (France *et al.*, 2000; Henslin, 2001; Liamputtong, 2007).

Participants in sensitive research who reveal highly personal and intimate details about their lives are vulnerable in a number of ways (Brannen, 1988; Demi & Warren, 1995; James & Platzer, 1999; Renzetti & Lee, 1993). They may be vulnerable to their own emotions being stirred by taking part in the research (Barnard, 2005; Hess, 2006; Paradis, 2000; Sin, 2005; Sque, 2000). Those who take part in research and disclose details of their private lives (especially women) may also be at risk from their partners (Bergen, 1993). Participants may be made vulnerable by the way the results of the research are presented and interpreted. This is a particularly important issue when the research is undertaken with a vulnerable or stigmatized group of people. Sensitive researchers need to be vigilant in ensuring that the results of the research are not used in such a way that further stigmatizes or marginalizes the group under study (Liamputtong, 2007).

Nevertheless, there are also some positive outcomes in participating in sensitive research. The research participants may find that by participating in a research project they are able to talk about matters that they might not otherwise have a chance to in every daylife or to anyone else (Cutcliffe & Ramcharan, 2002; Dyregrov, 2004; Gair, 2002; Grinyer, 2004; Hall & Kuilg, 2004; Hess, 2006; Liamputtong, 2007; Morse, 2000). The confidential nature of research that sensitive researchers ensure to the participants may permit these people to open up their concerns. For some people, participating in research provides them with a therapeutic experience (Cutcliffe & Ramcharan, 2002; Hess, 2006; Morse & Field, 1995; Norris, Nurius & Dimeff, 1996; Parris, Du Mont & Gombay, 2005; Usher & Holmes, 1997). And in some cases, it can be an empowering experience (Campbell, 2002; Rickard, 2003). People feel that at last someone listens to their vulnerable stories and for many, this gives them a chance to 'put it all together' (Baker, Lavende & Tincello, 2005; Dyregrov, 2004; Gair, 2002; Grinyer, 2004; Morse & Field, 1995). Very often, these people have been waiting for someone who would be interested in their stories (see Gair, 2002). John Cutcliffe and Paul Ramcharan (2002:1003) contend that although participation in research can bring up some painful feelings, 'it is also possible that telling their story can be therapeutic for the participants and thus could be regarded as producing a positive outcome for them, that is, a beneficent act'.

Legal issues

Researchers undertaking research on sensitive topics may be faced by some legal issues (Liamputtong, 2007). For example, researchers investigating child abuse are bound under mandatory reporting rules to report any child abuse to the police (Morse & Field, 1995; Socolar, Runyan & Amata-Jackson, 1995; Steinberg, Pynoos, Goenjaan *et al.*, 1999). Researchers involved in this type of research are under obligation to inform potential participants of this as part of the informed consent procedure. The obligation to report may have an impact on accessing a sample.

When undertaking research on sensitive topics, such as prostitution, child abuse or drug taking, there is a possibility that participants may disclose some types of illegal behaviour (Ferrell & Hamm, 1998; Lee, 1993; Melrose, 2002; Volker, 2004). In addition to being privy to disclosure of illegal activities, researchers may be placed in danger throughout the research (Hammersley & Atkinson, 1983; Lee, 1995). There are examples of researchers being threatened by partners of women taking part in research on domestic violence (Bergen, 1993; Parker & Ulrich, 1990). Researchers need to be aware of the possibility of this happening and understand their obligations to the research participants and to themselves.

The data collected by researchers can be subpoenaed for use in court cases (Liamputtong & Ezzy, 2005). Although this is a possibility in all research, due to the nature of the data collected, it may be more probable in research on sensitive issues (Lee, 1993). The National Health and Medical Research Council (NHMRC) in Australia has recognized that issues like these may arise when undertaking qualitative research and have alerted researchers that they may be legally required to testify in court and 'mandatory reporting of information that has been revealed by a participant may be required' (NHMRC, 2002:132). We do not claim that this happens at all times, but there have been a number of reports of researchers' data being subpoenaed by the courts for use in court cases (Ferrell & Hamm, 1998; Scarce, 1994; Shaffir & Stebbins, 1991). Researchers can run the risk of being imprisoned if they fail to comply with court orders to supply research data (Scarce, 1994). Thus, sensitive researchers need to be aware of the possibility of this happening and ensure they have strategies in place to deal with it.

Summary

In this chapter, we have provided readers with some theoretical and methodological perspectives that we relied on in carrying out the research that this book is based on. We argue that there are different paradigms in the social sciences, but as the nature of our study was to explore the lived experiences of undertaking sensitive research among researchers who have worked with vulnerable people, the constructivist focusing on qualitative research was deemed suitable for our study. Hence, what we will present in the chapters that follow will be based on our qualitative research.

In this chapter, we also point to some ethical and moral issues in undertaking sensitive research. The intrusion into participants' lives is pertinent to sensitive research and we are well aware of this intrusion. However, as we have suggested, it was not possible for our work to rely on existing records or publications, or on observation. The nature of our inquiry rendered the methodology we adopted. But, we have ensured that our methodology was not too intrusive (although some readers may suggest that in-depth interviews are always intrusive). We believe the ethical and moral issues are more important in any sensitive research and we have pointed to many issues in this chapter. We conclude the chapter with a discussion on legal issues that researchers may have to deal with in undertaking sensitive research. And this is something that we need to be mindful of as it can have ill effect on our well-being as researchers.

Tutorial activities

In this chapter, we discuss issues relating to methodological, theoretical, ethical and moral perspectives in undertaking sensitive research. By now, we hope that readers are more familiar with our research framework and some ethical issues and able to address the following:

(a) Discuss the importance of qualitative research in doing sensitive research in comparison to quantitative methods, and suggest other methodological frameworks that might be useful.

(b) Why do sensitive researchers need to think carefully about ethical and moral issues in carrying out sensitive research? What will be the implications for our research participants, and ourselves as researchers, if we do not think carefully about these issues?

SUGGESTED READING

Daly, K. (2007). *Qualitative Methods for Family Studies and Human Development.* London: Sage Publications.

Denzin, N.K. & Lincoln, Y.S. (eds.) (2005). *Handbook of Qualitative Research,* (3rd edn). Thousand Oaks, CA: Sage Publications.

Hesse-Biber, S.N. & Yaiser, M.L. (eds.) (2004). *Feminist Perspectives on Social Research.* New York: Oxford University Press.

Israel, M. & Hay, I. (2006). *Research Ethics for Social Scientists: Between Ethical Conduct and Regulatory Compliance.* London: Sage Publications.

Kellehear, A. (1990). *Dying of Cancer: The Final Year of Life*. London: Harwood Academic Publishers.

Liamputtong, P. (2007). *Researching the Vulnerable: A Guide to Sensitive Research Methods*. London: Sage Publications.

Liamputtong, P. & Ezzy, D. (2005). *Qualitative Research Methods* (2nd edn). Melbourne: Oxford University Press.

Richardson, L. (1997). *Fields of Play: Constructing an Academic Life*. New Brunswick, NJ: Rutgers University Press.

Saks, M. & Allsop, J. (eds.) (2007). *Researching Health: Qualitative, Quantitative and Mixed Methods*. London: Sage Publications.

Willis, J.W. (2007). *Foundations of Qualitative Research: Interpretive and Critical Approaches*. London: Sage Publications.

3

Conducting a sensitive research project

Data collection can be an intense experience, especially if the topic that one has chosen has to do with the illness experience or other stressful human experiences. The stories that the qualitative researcher obtains in interviews will be stories of intense suffering, social injustices, or other things that will shock the researcher.

(Morse & Field, 1995:78)

In this chapter we discuss the conduct and process of undertaking qualitative research on sensitive topics and raise some important points for researchers to consider throughout the research process. There are a number of specific issues regarding the process of entering people's lives for research purposes. These include rapport development, researcher self-disclosure, listening to untold stories, feelings of guilt and vulnerability, leaving the research relationship and researcher exhaustion. Data transcription and analysis are important phases in the qualitative research process and often require an enormous time commitment from researchers. In this chapter we will outline some of the difficulties faced by researchers from the time they enter into the lives of their participants through to data collection, transcription and analysis.

Entering the lives of others

In an examination of the experience of undertaking sensitive health research, it is important to first consider what it is that we, as qualitative researchers, actually do. We go into other people's lives, sometimes at a time of crisis and stress, and we ask them to talk in detail about their experiences (Cannon, 1992; Glesne & Peshkin, 1992; Liamputtong, 2007; Liamputtong & Ezzy, 2005; Morse & Field, 1995; Ribbens & Edwards, 1998). Sometimes this can be for an extended period of time involving repeated interviews, or it may be a one-off encounter.

As highlighted in Chapters 1 and 2, many researchers of sensitive topics choose a qualitative design using the in-depth interview as their preferred method of data collection. There are a range of issues that arise when qualitative interviewing is used by researchers investigating sensitive topics. One of the main issues raised is that these interviews are often stressful for both the researcher and the interviewee (Alty & Rodham, 1998; Burr, 1995; Campbell, 2002; Dunn, 1991; Gilbert, 2001b). In-depth interviews can be done on a one-off basis or they can involve a more longitudinal design with data collection and contact with participants extending over a period of time. The intensity and duration of the relationship will vary with the different methodologies and theoretical frameworks used to design the research.

Whether qualitative researchers plan their research around a single encounter with participants, or alternatively prioritize developing trust and rapport over a number of encounters is a contentious issue. Those in favour of one-off encounters state that participants will be more likely to disclose more to a researcher under such conditions (Brannen, 1988) along similar lines to the logic that anonymous surveys of sensitive topics illicit more honest responses (Clifford, 1997). Some of the researchers that we interviewed acknowledged that their participants often share private information about certain aspects of their lives that they would not normally expect to hear due to their status as a stranger,

Occasionally it's the first opportunity to do it and a stranger is always a good person to do it with the first time because there are no repercussions, or no obvious repercussions and that's important.

People talk about hurts that are years and years old that they haven't shared with anyone, cause often the people around them all have the wrong qualifications to share and I think one of the great things about being a researcher in this area is being a nobody.

Previous research has acknowledged that this lack of a relationship often makes it easier for people to open up and disclose personally sensitive information (Brannen, 1988; Reinharz, 1992). Often researchers do reassure their participants that the interview will be a one-off encounter, which may heighten disclosure. Daphne Patai (1991:142) raises the point that, as researchers:

we ask of the people we interview the kind of revelation of their inner life that normally occurs in situations of great familiarity and within the private realm. Yet we invite these revelations to be made in the context of the public sphere, which is where, in an obvious sense, we situate ourselves when we appear with tape recorders and note pads eager to promote our 'projects' for which other people are to provide the living matter.

During the decision-making process it is also important to consider the ethics and impact of the research encounter on the participant. That is, whether it is exploitive to establish a relationship with a research participant in order to encourage them to disclose more information (Oakley, 1981). This view is not supported by Sally Hutchinson and colleagues (1994) who believe that people who cannot tolerate talking about a sensitive topic simply will not do so. However, if the researcher is able to build a relationship with the participant

> **Box 3.1** Advantages and disadvantages of one-off encounters versus multiple contacts when conducting qualitative research on sensitive topics
>
> One-off encounters:
> - participants are more likely to reveal sensitive information due to the 'anonymity' of the encounter
> - researchers may be less likely to become emotionally involved or experience friendship–professional blurring of boundaries
> - may be more ethically correct for participants
> - are less likely to raise challenges in ending the relationship.
>
> Multiple contact research:
> - allows more time and opportunity for the development of rapport with the participant, which may in turn lead to increased disclosure
> - may be criticized as being exploitive of participants
> - increases the risk of boundary blurring for the researcher
> - may introduce challenges in ending the relationship with the research participant.

based on reciprocity and personal involvement then this may impact on their willingness to take part in the research and open a part of themselves that they ordinarily would keep closed. Some participants may not be aware of issues that taking part in research on a sensitive topic may evoke (Ramos, 1989). Research participants often do reveal highly personal aspects of their lives to researchers, which are beyond what people would normally disclose. While it is not possible to state whether one type of interview is better than another, it is important to note that the quality of the data collected may be dependent on the researcher's ability to develop an intimate and ongoing relationship with the participant. Box 3.1 summarizes some of the advantages and disadvantages of one-off encounters versus multiple contact research on sensitive topics.

Some of the researchers that we interviewed acknowledged that entering into the lives of others is characteristic of this type of research, suggesting that it is this aspect that makes the research unique.

I think, sort of generally, the idea of being allowed into people's lives is a real characteristic of the research that I do and it's, it's probably the most rewarding part of the research.

It is so much more than just signing a form to say that they are willing to offer you information, they are actually allowing you into their lives, they are telling you personal information that might be quite hard, so you need to demonstrate a certain degree of discretion, of respect, of appreciation for what they are doing cause the reality is that it is more than just words, it's more than just what you are going to analyze, it's their life, their experience and you need to make sure that you are aware of that.

Developing rapport

Regardless of whether the research involves a one-off encounter or multiple contacts, qualitative researchers must initiate a rapport-building process from their first encounter with a participant in order to build a research relationship that will allow the researcher access to that person's story (Ceglowski, 2000; Goodwin, Pope, Mort et al., 2003; Grbich, 1999; Liamputtong, 2007; Minichiello et al., 2000; Payne, 1994; Taylor & Bogdan, 1998). While the development of rapport is important for all qualitative research, creating and maintaining a rapport is one of the most important aspects of data collection in an in-depth interview on a sensitive topic (Johnson & Clarke, 2003; Lee, 1993; Taylor & Bogdan, 1998). There are a number of different strategies researchers can use to facilitate the development of good rapport and these are summarized in Box 3.2.

As stated by Victor Minichiello and colleagues (2000:179):

If we accept that in-depth interviewing necessitates establishing and maintaining good rapport with informants then it should also be recognised that such a process is never devoid of some form of emotional commitment from both sides of the fence.

Emotional commitment to the research may result in the researcher experiencing feelings of guilt when the relationship comes to an end (Burr, 1995; Cannon, 1989). Others have spoken about the difficulties faced by researchers

---

Box 3.2 Strategies to enhance rapport development between researchers and participants

- matching personal communication styles of the participant (language, speech patterns, tone, breathing patterns, posture etc.) (Minichiello, Aroni, Timewell et al., 2000)
- making an effort to get to know the lives of the participants (Berk & Adams, 2001)
- interviewing people in their own homes (where possible) (Taylor & Bogdan, 1998)
- making conversation with the participant prior to the interview (Liamputtong & Ezzy, 2005)
- having cups of tea or sharing a meal (Matocha, 1992)
- showing an active interest in the life of the person (e.g. looking at photos or the garden) (Miller & Tewksbury, 2001)
- active listening (Liamputtong & Ezzy, 2005; Minichiello, Madison, Hays et al., 1999).

when the participants in their studies die (Beaver *et al.*, 1999; Cannon, 1989, 1992; De Raeve, 1994). Researchers need to be able to prepare themselves to physically and emotionally disengage at the end of the research. Minichiello *et al.* (2000:174) report that very few researchers prepare themselves to exit 'and even fewer report on the process when providing details of their project'.

Some of the researchers interviewed spoke candidly about struggling with the level of rapport that they developed.

You need to just be able to sit and talk and develop a rapport with people because I think when that happens and I suppose in that way it's sort of a friendship because you do take the time when you get there to chat about things, have a cup of tea and then you sort of get ready for the interview.

I knew that it would be really important to develop rapport so that they could tell me all of these personal things so I was probably conscious of making sure that I had developed really strong well founded relationships with them but probably not thinking about the implications of that and the consequences of doing that.

Part of the role of the qualitative researcher is to facilitate participant disclosure. This disclosure can be heightened if there is a level of rapport between researcher and participant. Concern has been raised by a number of feminist authors regarding the level of disclosure achieved in some research interviews (Finch, 1984; Liamputtong, 2007; Oakley, 1981; Reinharz, 1992). Kvale (1996:116) echoes this point stating that the 'interviewer should also be aware that the openness and intimacy of the interview may be seductive and lead subjects to disclose information that they may later regret'.

Some of the researchers that we interviewed reported feeling quite surprised at the depth of information offered to them from their participant and that the act of listening to the story often validated the experiences of the participants by giving them the time to talk about their own experiences:

I am just amazed at how willing people were to talk to me about the most intimate and personal details of their lives.

. . . it's about respectfully listening to someone's story without comment; it's about listening to them and affirming the story by the listening.

In contrast, some of the other researchers interviewed felt a little uneasy about the level of disclosure that occurs in some research interviews.

Sometimes when people open up and tell their story they get carried away and before you know it they have told you about things that you wouldn't expect, that makes me feel a little uncomfortable at times.

Often qualitative research interviews take place in people's homes and people are effectively volunteering to allow researchers to come into a private part of their lives. When a researcher spends time developing rapport with a participant they may feel obliged to stay on for a while after the interview and spend some time with the participant.

I sometimes feel like perhaps just on the littlest level that they might feel that you are a friend and you feel a teeny bit guilty cause they are giving you cups of tea and being really nice and you are always thinking – 'Oh I am just getting my data here' but then again I always think that you have a responsibility to act in that socially acceptable way.

It is common for qualitative researchers to report on context, often taking detailed field notes about the setting of the interview. This may include observations of photographs of family members, descriptions of the house, the room, the person and pets. The researchers we interviewed often reported staying with the participants for a while after the completion of the interview, having a cup of tea, or taking a walk in the garden. While these courtesies are often important for rapport maintenance they may also create an expectation that the research relationship becomes more like a friendship.

You need to allow about half an hour before you even start talking about what you are there to talk about and then you can't just get up and leave, you've got to have afternoon tea and I felt I really needed to do that so that they could open up to me and so they didn't see me as someone – 'well she's just here to get the gory, gutsy bits and that's it'. I wanted to make sure that they knew how important it was for me to see them as a woman and to understand their context, like their life and the other parts.

Self-disclosure

Researcher self-disclosure or reciprocal sharing of personal stories, is a strategy that can be used by researchers to assist in the process of interviewing, particularly on sensitive topics (Liamputtong, 2007). In order to build a relationship with a participant so that they feel comfortable in telling their story, researchers may undertake a level of self-disclosure, for example, by sharing that they have a history of domestic abuse. As Oakley (1981:41) succinctly puts it:

In most cases, the goal of finding out about people through interviewing is best achieved when the relationship of interviewer to interviewee is non-hierarchical and when the interviewer is prepared to invest his or her own personal identity in the relationship.

Many of the researchers we interviewed spoke about undertaking a reciprocal sharing of personal stories as a way of ensuring that the relationship between themselves and the participant was non-hierarchical. Researcher self-disclosure was reportedly used by some researchers to create a 'level playing field', acknowledging that doing this may enhance rapport, show respect for the participants and validate their stories.

I needed to put myself on a level playing field with them in terms of – I think, as much as anything, make them understand that I really understand what they are going through – cause how many say 'oh yeah, I know what you mean', when they really don't . . . and I think I really wanted them to realize that I understood.

All of my questions and my inquiries and conversations are highly personal, so there's no way I can expect not to be asked to be on a level playing field with those people, they are going to ask me and they do and that's fine. I'm not one of those people who has too much of a problem with that. I'm happy to talk about any personal aspect of my life – most of the time.

Although many qualitative researchers undertake some level of disclosure in research interviews, the intensity and frequency of disclosure may be different in research on sensitive topics (Lee, 1993; Lee & Renzetti, 1993). There was recognition by the researchers we interviewed that qualitative research on sensitive topics creates a space for self-disclosure by the researchers that may not be appropriate in other types of research.

I expect to be sharing in a way with those people. What happens is that when people talk to me about their experiences they share with me and I share with them, it's much more of an equal relationship than a conventional research interview.

Some of the researchers we interviewed described how they went through a process of mentally preparing themselves for undertaking some level of self-disclosure in the interview. In contrast there were others who had not thought about it too much, and had to then make a decision on the spur of the moment about how much to share.

I was in an interview where suddenly I had to make a decision about disclosure – and this is not just disclosure about what my schooling was or you know what my parents did, this was a very, very intimate moment of disclosure and I told him and he said – 'that's the same as mine'.

I suddenly realised that if you are going to go into this kind of work where you are getting into very, very intimate questions with people you have to be prepared to give something – you can't play the objective researcher.

I didn't want to [disclose personal information], no I didn't. Not that I was disappointed cause I got to the point where I thought well if that's what's had to happen for me to feel like I connect, because for some women that was quite important and also it was like it was coming out of my mouth before I even realized it and it felt like I had no sense of control because I wanted her to know that I identified with her and I wanted her to know that I knew what it was like.

Others researchers spoke about how they actively planned about the level of disclosure they felt comfortable with before they undertook the interview.

The principle is disclose as little as possible and always disclose the minimum amount if you have to, to get where you need to go.

I knew that because it was such a sensitive issue that I had to lay myself on the table – literally.

Some researchers spoke about feeling that their research participants did not want to hear about them, often reminding themselves that this was not about the researcher but about those who were participating.

. . . you know it's an interview and not a sharing session, hopefully they've understood what it's about and you know I avoid talking about me.

I think I'm always thinking that no-one wants to hear about me when I'm here to hear about them.

I constantly remind myself that this is not about me, although sometimes it could be, this is about her and her experience.

While it appeared that some researchers felt quite comfortable with a certain level of disclosure, for others it seemed to create some angst, especially for those who had made a decision before going into the interview not to self-disclose.

For God's sake – you've just set yourself up to say that you are not gonna do this and this and you've walked out of this woman's house for the first time and you've told her everything about yourself, you know? And I've sort of thought, 'Oh God, does that make me a bad researcher?' because I'm there to find out about her but all of a sudden I'm talking just as much about me as she's telling me about herself.

I sort of felt quite hot and flustered and was quite taken aback and I'm still trying to listen to what this man is telling me but thinking, like sitting there, nodding and saying yes and listening to him on a superficial level and thinking 'oh shit, oh shit, I've just compromised myself, I've just done what I said I wouldn't do'.

Researcher self-disclosure is often reported as good research practice, particularly by feminist writers (Liamputtong, 2007; Oakley, 1981; Reinharz, 1992). Despite the fact that it may be used by researchers as a way of 'levelling the field', it can sometimes make researchers feel vulnerable. It is important for researchers to be aware of the potential consequences of disclosure and it may be helpful to think through how much self-disclosure they will undertake prior to the interview (Fontana & Frey, 1994; Oakley, 1981). Strategies for research self-protection are discussed in more detail in Chapter 7.

Reciprocity

Closely linked with researcher self-disclosure is reciprocity. Qualitative research on a sensitive topic needs to run on the principles of 'fair exchange' (Daly, 1992:5) whereby a researcher and participant engage in a reciprocal sharing process (Acker, Barry & Essevald, 1991). This reciprocal sharing may be related to a sharing of disclosure whereby researcher and participant share aspects of their stories with each other, or it might relate to a situation where a researcher becomes involved in other aspects of a participants' life (such as running errands or providing help with childcare) with the aim that this will contribute to the depth and quality of the data. While this reciprocity can reduce the hierarchical nature of the research process, it may also leave a researcher feeling that they need to 'give something back' to the participants. Giving back in this way, may enable researchers to acknowledge the value of what the participants have shared with them. As Claire Wenger contends, 'there needs to be giving as well as receiving in these exchanges' (Wenger, 2002:272). Sarah Goodrum and Jennifer Keys (2007:255) offered three types of reciprocity in their study examining the experiences of losing a loved one to murder and the termination of a pregnancy: financial compensation, interpersonal exchanges and follow-up contacts.

Some of the researchers that we interviewed shared their thoughts about reciprocity.

I'm not gonna hold back and not offer myself to them as a source of support just, just to make sure that my research is within the confines of what a textbook says – like this is a real experience for them, they are letting me into their lives, they're – you know – privileging me so I actually need to give them something back.

I am here doing research but because I have been able to offer you advice, or because I have been able to sit and spend time with you, then isn't that equally important as what you actually are offering me . . . I think it really is a reciprocal thing, it was totally a two-way street.

I think reciprocity is really important in all relationships and as a researcher it is a relationship, limited and contrived though it is, there are still kind of certain rules that you follow – they give you something, you give them something back.

It can't be a 'slam bam thank you ma'am' situation, you go there and you expect that you will be required to give something.

Differing understandings and levels of reciprocity were reported by the researchers we interviewed. Some were related directly to the research, while others related more closely to a social relationship with the participant. Some of the researchers reported that their reciprocity took the form of some community action, a report or some community service. For others, it was about offering more tangible support such as running errands or going out to a movie or a dinner with the participant. Similarly, differing understandings of reciprocity have been reported in the literature with some writers advising strongly against reciprocal relationships (Acker *et al.*, 1991; Stacey, 1988) while others (particularly feminist writers) advocating strongly for research relationships based on reciprocity (Cotterill, 1992; Ribbens & Edwards, 1998; Stanley, 1990; Stanley & Wise, 1991). One of the most important aspects of undertaking research based on feminist principles is the acknowledgement of the links between emotion and knowledge (Campbell, 2002; DeVault, 1997; Ellis, 1991; Fonow & Cook, 1991; Jaggar, 1989; Kleinman & Copp, 1993; Krieger, 1991; Wilkins, 1993). In addition to the acknowledgement of emotion, feminist researchers often advocate for the development of relationships based on reciprocity and sharing (Acker *et al.*, 1991; Oakley, 1998). Joan

Acker, Kate Barry and Johanna Essevald (1991:41) have recognized that research relationships developed in this way can be problematic, stating that 'often this meant that our relationship was defined as something which existed beyond the limits of the interview situation'. Difficulties with disengaging from the research relationships have been articulated by a number of authors (Burr, 1995; Cannon, 1989; Hubbard, Backett-Milburn & Kemmer, 2001; Ridge *et al.*, 1999; Rowling, 1999; Russell, 1999; Scott, 1998) and will be discussed in more detail in the following chapter.

Being human and caring

Throughout the interviews, researchers identified a number of important considerations that need to be taken into account when undertaking qualitative research interviews. While it could be argued that many of these reflect good qualitative research practice, generally they have been identified as particularly important in the conduct of sensitive research interviews, especially interviews that involve potentially vulnerable participants (Liamputtong, 2007). The issues identified included being human and caring, listening supportively and actively, and showing emotion and empathy (for more detail see Grbich, 1999; Liamputtong & Ezzy, 2005; Minichiello *et al.*, 2000; Morse, 1997).

Many of the researchers we interviewed spoke about the fact that the people participating in their research were often marginalized and vulnerable and some researchers felt that participation in research provided an opportunity for some people to be listened to by a person who really did want to hear their story.

A lot of women were saying that they actually look forward to me coming because it was almost like their time, to talk about personal things, things that they don't often get to talk about, especially to someone who really wants to listen.

Qualitative researchers attempt to access the 'human story' and in order to do this it is important to remember the human side of the work. Qualitative research is:

. . . so different because people are giving us something, they are giving us their words, a part of themselves.

In recounting their experiences, many of the researchers we interviewed spoke about the need to be human and not being scared to show human emotions as this often facilitated the research process and was good research practice.

You have to appear real and human in this research, be honest, be caring and think about the person, the human person when you are writing it up.

It wasn't just being passed to a tape recorder, it was information being given to me as a human being and I responded to them as a human being.

When this researcher talked about 'responding as a human being' she referred to her ability to care for another person. A number of conceptualizations of caring have been developed by different theorists (Leininger, 1981; Morse, Botorff, Neander et al., 1991; Morse, Solberg, Neander et al., 1990; Noddings, 1984); however, many theorists who conceptualize caring as a human trait claim that caring is a part of human nature (i.e. one of those things that makes us human). Jan Morse and colleagues (1990:4) state that, caring is 'an innate human trait, the human mode of being, a part of human nature, and essential to human existence'. In this sense, caring is perceived to be a basic characteristic that is a foundation of human science (Leininger, 1981; Roach, 1987; Van Hooft, 1995). Caring as a human trait has been widely explored by Martin Heidegger (1962) who asserts that caring is a way of being in the world in which people and things matter. Heidegger's analysis led him to conclude that one of the most basic components of being in the world (being human) is the experience of *sorge* or care (Heidegger, 1962).

Caring as a concept is discussed in detail, particularly in the nursing literature (Morse et al., 1991; Morse et al., 1990; Noddings, 1984; Roach, 1987) and there are parallels for researchers. If caring is a basic human trait, then it is vital that researchers are able to care for another person during the research process. Nel Noddings (1984), a noted nursing caring theorist, calls for professional practice grounded in caring and highlights that caring for another involves 'a desire for the other's well-being' and a 'commitment of self' to others (Noddings, 1984:13). Caring for a person implies that we are willing to be available and to give something of ourselves to others, and it sometimes involves a level of guilt (Noddings, 1984).

Caring theorists have identified a number of behaviours that they see as essentially 'caring' ones. Madeleine Leininger (1981:13) uses the following terms to illustrate some of the behaviours that may be expected when a person is involved in caring for another: 'comfort, compassion, concern, coping behaviour, empathy, enabling, facilitating, interest, involvement, sharing, support, tenderness, touching and trust'. An examination of these terms suggests that researchers involved in qualitative research working on sensitive topics are engaged in many of these behaviours as a result of the research that they do. The researchers we interviewed referred to themselves as caring, empathetic, patient and compassionate. They also reflected on the value of just being with a participant, especially when the participant was disclosing something particularly intimate to the researcher.

When he became so upset I switched the tape recorder off and in doing this there was a real shift to the personal. I stopped being a researcher and I became another person in the room with him, I gave him a hug, we had a cigarette – it was much more human.

One of the important aspects of this discussion is that 'if we undertake to study human lives, we have to be ready to face human feelings' (Ely, Anzul,

Friedman *et al.*, 1991:49), which often comes at a personal cost to researchers. Some of the researchers talked frankly about the importance of responding to the participants as human beings. They spoke about the value of touching, offering support, showing emotion and generally 'being with' the participant while they told their story.

One researcher shared her concerns regarding touching participants, recounting a time when she had reached out and held the hand of the participant while she was telling her story. She felt confused and concerned afterwards because she felt that when she did reach out and hold the hand of the other person, there was a shift in the relationship.

When I held her hand I thought 'hey, hang on – the dimensions have changed here, the line between me as a friend and me as a researcher may be blurred because – is that appropriate researcher conduct?'

The blurring of boundaries is of significant concern to qualitative researchers involved in research on sensitive topics and will be explored in more detail in the following chapter.

Untold stories

In order for researchers to understand the experiences of participants, they need to build a level of trust so that the participant feels safe enough to share their story (Booth & Booth, 1994; Charmaz, 1991). Given that some of these stories may never have been shared before, this is not always an easy process. When a research participant feels that they are in a safe place they may feel more inclined to share some aspects of their lives that they may not have shared previously. Many of the researchers that were interviewed spoke about providing a safe place for people to tell their story.

The participants feel safe because there is a huge level of trust there and it is like an invitation to them to talk about all those sorts of issues and there won't be any repercussions for them.

I was almost like a safe place, it was almost like I was an opportunity to vent all of their inner fears, their really raw emotions that they weren't prepared to give to other people cause they were trying to protect those other people whereas I was there and happy to take, seen as almost happy to take all that on board.

I was viewed as a safe place and yeah I think that they had talked about things with other people to a certain level but maybe not enough for them to be satisfied.

Although there is a recognition that providing a space for people to talk is an important feature of qualitative research, Daphne Patai (1991) has identified that many people who participate in research do not have enough people in their lives who want to listen to what they have to say. This concern has been echoed by Margaret Ely and her colleagues (1991) who raised a concern that some people who do not have many opportunities to talk about their experiences might take advantage of the opportunity to participate in a research interview.

Many of the stories that are told in research interviews are the ones that participants have kept hidden from family and friends in order to protect them. When we invite participants to tell their stories it is important to allow them to tell that story in their own way.

. . . so the untold stories are often about being given permission to talk about the topics that you are not really supposed to talk about and being given permission by someone who wants to know, someone who you hope will be a bit impartial and unbiased will listen and whose job isn't to solve a problem but just to listen.

For many participants in research on sensitive topics, it is the first time that they have told someone their story, and this can raise difficulties not only for them, but also for the researcher who is listening to the story. This sharing of hidden or unexplored aspects of people's lives can change the expectations of the participants. The fact that qualitative research often requires supportive listening may make researchers ultimately more vulnerable to crossing the boundaries from research into friendship.

Many of the stories that qualitative researchers hear are private ones that participants had not yet shared.

You don't want the public face, you want the private face of the sensitive issue cause the public face is what everyone thinks is okay to talk about whereas if you are going to research in sensitive topics you actually want what people are not talking about publicly.

People talk about and reveal aspects of themselves to me that normally would remain unexamined all together or private . . . sometimes it can be like opening up Pandora's box, you never know what you are going to get.

Some of it is the relief of telling someone . . . just anyone – they don't want to die with their secrets inside them.

In the process of undertaking a research interview, researchers are often privy to these stories for a number of reasons (Etherington, 1996; Ramos, 1989; Wincup, 2001). As outlined in Chapter 1, Michelle Ramos (1989) terms this the 'Pandora's box' phenomenon illustrating that in qualitative research we often ask people to talk about aspects of their lives that they may not have previously discussed. In a similar vein, Kim Etherington (1996) uses the term 'tin-opener effect' to illustrate the fact that qualitative research can take people to places where they may not want to go.

Many of those interviewed reported worrying about the effects of opening up 'Pandora's box' or a 'can of worms', not only for the participants but for themselves.

I think that we are opening up a can of worms. People do open up and sometimes tell things that I don't think they have really thought through.

I chatted to her and she ended up telling me how she'd fallen in love with her husband and it was quite funny and we were just sitting in the huge waiting queue and we had heaps of time and she said to me – 'it's so funny, I've only just met you and I've told you this whole story' and that was really nice.

As part of this process, the researcher may then also become a secret-keeper. For some researchers interviewed, the role of secret-keeper was not one that they felt entirely comfortable with.

I had to keep that secret and you know I didn't like being a keeper of secrets but I'd set the study up so I could get the secrets and so I had to deal with that.

I am compelled to keep those secrets and that is a big responsibility.

Researchers listening to those secrets often felt that they were somehow performing a service for the participant, likening the experience to that of hearing a religious confession.

. . . people discuss their sexual problems with me, and some people will tell me something they felt guilty about for 40 years, and some people will confess their sins or what they consider to be sins – something they have kept secret for a long time and felt sad about and they will trust this secret to me.

Researchers might create a confessional situation for participants by openly inviting them to tell their story. This may provide an opportunity for a person to confess something that may be particularly difficult to tell anyone outside of that situation (Lupton, 1998). Deborah Lupton (1998:92) suggests that 'the confession is deemed to be a difficult but rewarding process', acknowledging that people can feel purified by the process of telling another. Thus, confessions can provide a sense of catharsis. The cathartic effects of research have been well documented in the literature with many authors commenting on the perceived benefits of participating in research interviews (Brannen, 1993; Hutchinson *et al.*, 1994; Sque, 2000).

Feeling privileged

Many of the researchers we interviewed used the term 'privilege' when describing their experiences. They often felt that they had been afforded a privilege by being allowed to listen to stories that were often private and intimate.

I suppose when it first happened I was very aware of the weight of the privilege of what I had been told.

. . . it is an enormous privilege for people to share the story of their life with you.

I think one needs to . . . go in with an awareness that first of all it is a privilege to be there and secondly that these are human beings, not research subjects.

The privilege of participating in this type of research has been documented in the literature (Cannon, 1992; Liamputtong Rice & Ezzy, 1999; Rosenblatt & Fischer, 1993; Sullivan, 1998). Kate Sullivan (1998:74), in her vivid description of her experiences when interviewing people whose partners had died states, 'at the forefront of my mind was always the thought that to be permitted a private view of another person's past, their pain, and their sorrow, was a privilege'. Qualitative researchers often feel that they are being made privy to privileged information, which may leave them with a heavy responsibility (Rosenblatt & Fischer, 1993). Researchers report coming away from research interviews with feelings of 'gratitude and debt to the person who has just shared many intimate details of their life' (Liamputtong Rice & Ezzy, 1999:41).

The privilege of being allowed access to an intimate story also meant that many researchers interviewed felt a sense of responsibility to 'do something' with that story.

. . . it is more than just signing a form to say that they are willing to offer you information, they are actually allowing you into their lives, they are telling you personal information that might be quite hard so you need to demonstrate a certain degree of discretion, of respect, of appreciation for actually what they are doing because the reality is that it is more than just words, it's more than just what you are going to analyze – it's their life, their experience and you need to make sure that you are aware of that.

But with the privilege of access comes awesome responsibility.

There is a bit of a responsibility that goes with listening to someone's story, especially when you know that they haven't told anyone before.

For some, the responsibility of being given the story weighed heavily on their conscience, leaving them with the feeling that failing to do something to help that person's situation would be letting that person down.

I have an incredible responsibility, I've been given this and I have to do something with it. I really felt a sense that I would be letting those people down if I did not and . . . I guess because we do come to know them through their stories this can have an effect on us.

Part of the responsibility felt by some of the researchers related to the fact that they were dealing with human lives and human feelings. Some reflected on the need to remember the human side when you are analyzing the data so that you remember that you do have a responsibility to treat both the data and the person with respect.

Remember that individual, that human being, when you are writing about them and imagine that human being reading what you have written and it's a heavy responsibility.

I'm saying that you have a responsibility to these people both in what you do with the information that they give you and what you do with them. I think it is extraordinarily rude to conduct an interview and then never have any contact with that person again.

Others expressed a need to follow-up the interview with a phone call or some other contact that reflected to the participants the importance of their participation in the project.

I've been fairly careful to take a note of it at the time [upcoming medical appointment or anniversary of death], put it in my diary and the day before or the day after ring them up and ask them how it was going . . . not necessarily as part of the research but just because I felt that I had a responsibility to them – they had told all this and it would be awful for them to tell somebody this and the person they were telling not to think that it was important.

Becoming desensitized

A number of the researchers we interviewed used the term *desensitization* when recounting their experiences. This feeling of becoming desensitized stemmed from the fact that they had heard so many difficult stories throughout their research careers that they did not get affected by them anymore.

. . . it's like those sorts of things just wear off, you know you don't get a shock when someone says – oh my father beat me for ten years, you just think 'oh well'.

One researcher felt that undertaking the research had an inoculation effect on her and that she would become immune to being shocked by the difficulties faced by some people.

I think towards the end there I started to worry about that sort of inoculation effect you know – after you've done it so many times and you've heard so many bad stories – do you become immune to it?

Concerns over desensitization have also been raised by many other authors (Campbell, 2002; Melrose, 2002; Morgan & Krone, 2001; Scott, 1998). Sara Scott (1998:22) explains that often throughout interview discussions of rape, physical assault and childhood prostitution – the extraordinary can become 'bizarrely ordinary'. This anxiety has been echoed among health workers who found similar concerns in medical students who reported being anxious about becoming desensitized and estranged from their feelings (Smith & Kleinman, 1989). Although many of the researchers we interviewed did not have the extended contact with people that medical professionals do, their concerns about becoming distant from their feelings are important. Becoming estranged from your feelings is one of the responses to stress that has been reported in the literature that may have health damaging effects (Pearlman, 1995; Zapf, Seifert, Schmutte *et al.*, 2001). Signs of burnout and other important health issues are discussed further in Chapter 5.

Developing attachments

Developing attachments to research participants emerged as a significant issue for many of the researchers we interviewed. Many of them reported developing emotional attachments to the people involved in their research.

. . . there's some sort of emotional attachment going on and so I knew that it would happen and for a couple of people that I interviewed, well they developed an attachment to me which I had, I had to deal with.

Sometimes it became more like a friendship:

. . . she sort of has become a friend – we've chatted about lots of things . . . like we go out for dinner and I've chatted to her on the phone like um – when she's had a doctor's appointment I've rung her and said 'oh how did it go?' and when she had the last appointment I rang her and it was really upsetting for me cause the doctor said well we can't do anything for you at all and I got off the phone and I cried and I've got a meeting with her on Friday and that's going to be hard because I really do know her more as a person than just someone that I go and visit.

Many researchers interviewed commented about developing friendship-like relationships with research participants that raised issues about the boundaries in this type of research. Boundary blurring is discussed in more detail in the following chapter.

Researchers do continue to think about the people who participated in their research even after the data collection is completed. Undertaking the research process involves revisiting the data a number of times over the life of the project. One researcher spoke of her difficulty when reading through a draft report of her research that made her think again about those people who had been in her research.

I will never forget her as long as I live – she told me her story of being raped, a violent rape, so moving, so awful . . . the resilience of the human spirit. I can never forget her face, so young but yet so old. This research was about homelessness – I thought about what I might hear but I hadn't really prepared for that, for the horror of that story. How do you prepare for something like that?

Feeling vulnerable

Much of the literature regarding vulnerability in research focuses on the vulnerable nature of being a research subject but not on the researcher's vulnerability. Researcher vulnerability may be related to the setting of the research, particularly if the research is taking place in people's homes (Jamieson, 2000; Warr, 2004). Researchers in the current study reported feeling both physically and emotionally vulnerable.

You can feel vulnerable, one person that I interviewed turned out to have psychotic symptoms so I did feel a bit vulnerable in that situation, you do feel a bit vulnerable in that type of circumstance, you sort of feel unsafe or think gee what they are going to do.

I mean I have discovered my own vulnerability and considered it for the first time through these guys – it's really powerful.

You do feel vulnerable in research, to your own emotions. People are giving something of themselves and sometimes that affects you – as a person . . . who you are and how you do things.

Feelings of vulnerability for these researchers often came from the fact that in doing the research they were sometimes learning things about themselves. As Sandra Weber (1986:66) suggests, 'through dialogue, we get to think things through, glancing at the mirror the other holds up to us, discovering not only the other, but ourselves'. This point is echoed by Hans Gadamer (1995) who asserts that knowledge in the human sciences always has something of self-knowledge about it, which may give researchers a sense of their own vulnerability. In listening to a person's account of their life or their illness experience, we are effectively opening up in an embodied and personal way to the suffering of that other person, which may give us a heightened sense of our own mortality and vulnerability. Part of this vulnerability relates to an attempt by researchers to 'even up' the relationship between researcher and participant because if the participants are vulnerable then we too must be prepared to show our vulnerabilities (Stanley & Wise, 1993:177). Researchers may be vulnerable to their own emotions and experiencing that emotion may have effects on other aspects of their lives (Behar, 1996; Jamieson, 2000; Lankshear, 2000). Undertaking qualitative research can be a life-changing experience for some researchers, providing them with opportunities to assess certain aspects of their lives (Ellis, Kiesinger & Tillmann-Healy, 1997; Rosenblatt, 2001). Paul Rosenblatt (2001:124) echoes this point by saying:

. . . experiences interviewing individuals and families about heavy things in their lives have changed me as a human in relationship to other humans, have changed how I view myself and others.

Feeling guilty and the 'ethical hangover'

A number of researchers we interviewed expressed concern about feeling guilty about undertaking sensitive research interviews. For some, the feelings of guilt related to the interview process. Some were concerned about the effects of the research on the participants, while for others it related to feelings about the data that was being collected.

. . . and we ask them to give up a lot of their time and usually dredge up some really emotional stuff for them and then the best we can do is say 'oh well here's a phone number.'

It really does matter because they have opened up their chest and you rip bits out of them and then you just leave them with the wounds.

Some researchers felt like they were 'using' their participants as a means to an end. This feeling has also been articulated by Corrine Glense and Alan Peshkin (1992:112) who state that:

Questions of exploitation or 'using' others tend to arise as you become immersed in research and begin to rejoice in the richness of what you are learning. You are thankful, but instead of simply appreciating the gift, you may feel guilty for how much you are receiving and how little you are giving in return.

Researchers often get quite excited about the data that they are gathering but, at the same time, they grapple with feeling a little uncomfortable about what they are being told.

I mean this is a 14 year old and I don't even know if she is still alive and you are feeling somehow, not questioning your own morality but you just, at one level you know that this is good data, we've got two 14 year olds in our study, and you don't hopefully really think that because you are also thinking – this is shocking, there are 14 year olds on the street in this very vulnerable situation but at the same time you are happy to have gotten the information from them.

This idea of feeling excited by the data gathered but a little guilty about it has also been raised in the literature (Etherington, 1996; Finch, 1984; Lofland & Lofland, 1995; Oakley, 1981; Spalek, 2007). John Lofland and Lyn Lofland (1995:28) refer to this feeling as an 'ethical hangover', which is a 'feeling of persistent guilt or unease over what is viewed as a betrayal of the people under study'. Similarly, Kim Etherington (1996:347) reports her unease, 'as I listened to some of these stories with my 'researcher' ears, I became uncomfortable when I realized that I was thinking this is really good stuff!' For some researchers this sense of excitement when they obtain data from people is often in stark contrast with their ethics about using people for research purposes.

Exhaustion

Part of the investment of personal identity in the research relationship involves researchers taking their and their participants' emotions into account in the collection and interpretation of the data. This emotion can take the form of verbal and non-verbal communication. For example pauses, silences and non-verbal emotional displays such as tears and embarrassment also need to be included in the data set and analysis. While there has been acknowledgement that there needs to be an emotional commitment made by researchers and participants, the impacts of making such a commitment have not been well documented.

Many of the researchers we interviewed spoke about being emotionally and/or physically exhausted both during and after the research. For many of them, the sense of exhaustion came from the sheer number of interviews that they were required to do, and for others it was more about the content of the interviews.

. . . for me as an interviewer I guess I used to come away fairly exhausted, mentally exhausted, yeah just kind of like, a little worn out and incredibly grateful.

Emotional and physical exhaustion emerged as a major issue for researchers working on sensitive topics and will be further explored in Chapter 5.

Analyzing the data

There are a number of issues associated with the analysis and transcription of qualitative interview data. The goal of transcription is to transform oral speech into a printed copy, accurately capturing the words of the research participant (Sandelowski, 1994). Accurate transcription is the fundamental first step in data analysis. In order to undertake a transcription, researchers often listen to the interview tapes a number of times, becoming more familiar with the data on each listening. While some researchers opt to have their transcription of tapes performed by another person, most of the researchers interviewed preferred to undertake their own transcribing, believing that this was an important first step in the data analysis.

The process of transcription is often thought of as purely a technical task involving the transformation of the spoken word into data. The challenges associated with transcription have not been given a great deal of empirical attention. However, some researchers have acknowledged the difficulties associated with transcription of research interviews regarding sensitive topics (Cameron, 1993; Darlington & Scott, 2002; Etherington, 2007; Gair, 2002; Gilbert, 2001b; Gregory, Russell & Phillips, 1997; Lalor, Begley & Devane, 2006; McCosker, Barnard & Gerber, 2001; Melrose, 2002; Scott, 1998; Warr, 2004; Wray *et al.*, 2007). Transcribing a research interview on a sensitive topic can be an emotional experience for the transcriber who often listens to powerful stories. Transcribers are 'absorbing the voices and stories of research' (Warr, 2004:586), and they are often 'relistening to the suffering of research participants' (Wray *et al.*, 2007:1397); however, they are often overlooked when researchers think through the ethical issues that the research may raise. One of the researchers interviewed said:

Well I think that transcribing is kind of an overlooked process. I like to transcribe my own because I think by the time you have transcribed you know it really well and there is no substitute for that. To hear a voice is quite different to reading it on a page. You know a lot of people do send that kind of stuff out and never have a thought for what the transcriber, who has often not had anything much to do with the research, is going through.

Many of the researchers interviewed reported a range of difficulties associated with undertaking their own transcription of sensitive research interviews.

I do my own and it's one of the hardest aspects of this research, in the interview you hear what they say but when you listen again it's like, like you really hear it and you have time to take it in more . . . that's often the hardest bit.

Some of these difficulties related directly to the nature of the topic, and for others it was more about their own reactions to the data.

. . . cause you can hear the voice warbling and you can hear the silences and I can hear me, like sometimes at a silence – and my awkwardness and my uncomfortableness with the topic.

. . . it just broke my heart – I mean it broke my heart to hear the story and every time I came back to try and analyze that material it broke my heart.

Some researchers spoke about feeling quite emotional at the time of the transcription, and for some the transcription process allowed them the freedom to really respond emotionally to the data.

I have just read part of the transcript and I mean I felt much more emotional reading the transcript than what I had in the interview.

I find transcribing interviews really hard and its harder to transcribe the interview than it is to hear it the first time cause the second time you have to actually hear it and feel it.

I concede that with that I cried buckets when I did the transcription cause I didn't cry when I did the interviews. It was really sad and I'm sure that it all had accumulated interest and by the time I got to the transcription, when I was at home in my room with no-one else there, that's when I was able to do that kind of grieving for those who told such awful stories.

It has been suggested that ethics committees and institutional review committees could help to raise the awareness of the potential vulnerability of transcribers by including their role on application forms, which may help to protect transcribers (Dickson-Swift, James, Kippen *et al.*, 2008; Etherington, 2007; Gregory *et al.*, 1997). This is discussed further in Chapter 7.

Summary

Researchers undertaking research on sensitive topics do face a number of challenges throughout the research process. While some relate to the process of actually undertaking an interview, rapport building and use of self-disclosure, researchers also face ongoing challenges such as dealing with attachments, hearing untold stories, experiencing feelings of guilt, vulnerability and exhaustion, and issues related to both transcribing and analyzing qualitative data. At this stage, readers might be thinking that this all sounds fairly depressing and while we would agree that this can be a challenging process, there are many things that researchers *can* do to prepare themselves for challenges like these, which will be discussed in more detail in the chapters that follow.

Tutorial activities

(a) In this chapter we discussed the importance of developing rapport with research participants. Consider the scenario where you are planning to interview women who have suffered a miscarriage. What strategies might you instigate in order to enhance the development of rapport?

(b) We also discussed in this chapter the important skill of active listening. Work together with a classmate or colleague to practise your active listening skills. If you have access to a video camera you might like to record the mock interviews so that you can later critique your active listening skills. What specific indictors will you look for to assess quality active listening?

SUGGESTED READING

Dickson-Swift, V., James, E.L., Kippen, S. & Liamputtong, P. (2007). Doing sensitive research: what challenges do qualitative researchers face? *Qualitative Research*, **7**(3), 327–353.

Liamputtong, P. (2007). *Researching the Vulnerable: A Guide to Sensitive Research Methods*. London: Sage Publications.

Liamputtong, P. & Ezzy, D. (2005). *Qualitative Research Methods*. South Melbourne: Oxford University Press.

Morse, J.M. & Field, P.A. (1995). *Qualitative Research Methods for Health Professionals*. Thousand Oaks: Sage Publications.

4

Managing boundaries
in sensitive research

The uncertainty of where appropriate boundaries should lie is an ongoing concern in qualitative research and one that has received surprisingly little published attention, particularly from the lived perspective of the researcher.

(Gilbert, 2001a:4)

Qualitative health researchers immerse themselves in the settings that they are studying and this results in personal interaction with research participants. As a consequence of this immersion the boundaries between the researcher and the group of people under study can easily become 'blurred'. While many authors make fleeting references to some of the boundary issues they have experienced in their research (Birch & Miller, 2000; Campbell, 2002; Etherington, 1996; Gilbert, 2001a; Hutchinson & Wilson, 1994), very few have specifically examined the boundaries that arise for researchers and how they handle them. In this chapter we focus on the boundary issues inherent in sensitive research including boundaries between researcher/friend, researcher and counsellor/therapist and self/other. We conclude the chapter with a discussion of the implications of poor boundary management for researchers and outline some strategies that might be useful to researchers when managing these boundaries.

Defining boundaries

The term 'boundary' is used widely in the published literature, with most references to 'boundary blurring' found in clinical areas including counselling, psychotherapy, nursing and medicine. In very general terms the word boundary implies the determining of some type of limit or distance between persons (Scopelliti et al., 2004). The differing types of boundaries managed by counsellors, therapists and nurses have been well documented (Katherine, 1991; Walker & Clark, 1999; Webb, 1997); however, discussions of boundary issues faced by researchers are rare. One recent exception to this is the work of

Kathleen Gilbert (2001a:12) who argues that boundaries are an important aspect of qualitative research, particularly when researching sensitive topics. She states:

The combination of highly charged topics, an in-depth and long-term contact with the phenomenon and the evolving emotional environment of the researcher's own social world may result in a lack of clarity or 'fuzziness' in boundaries. These boundaries must be negotiated and renegotiated, an ongoing part of the research process, as a balance is sought between the dangers and benefits of being too far in or too far out of the lives of the researched.

Professional boundaries

The blurring of boundaries between being a healthcare professional and a researcher and the difficulties associated with remaining in a researcher role have been described (Hoddinott & Pill, 1997; Johnson & Clarke, 2003; Rager, 2005a, 2005b; Richards & Schwartz, 2002; Rowling, 1999). Many healthcare professionals are socialized into maintaining a sense of 'professional detachment' (Lupton, 1994), which enables them to maintain a safe boundary between themselves and their clients. Erving Goffman (1959) terms this 'role distancing' and it has been cited as a useful measure to address occupational stress in human service occupations particularly for social workers (Bennett, Evans & Tattersall, 1993). This distancing requires workers to be able to set clear boundaries between themselves and their clients or work situations (Lonne, 2003). These boundaries are thought to prevent the workers from becoming 'emotionally overwhelmed' (Lonne, 2003:293) by the often distressing situations that confront them. While this concept is useful for understanding how professionals manage boundaries it has not been fully explored in relation to researchers working on sensitive topics.

Many of the researchers we interviewed reported being concerned about the management of professional boundaries and referred to the need to distance themselves from the research, which often left them grappling with the idea of 'being professional'. For many, this included not getting emotionally involved in the research and being good at managing the boundaries.

I just thought that I was so professional that you know that wasn't going to happen [getting emotionally involved].

In spite of this, researchers, like other professionals, *do* experience a certain level of emotional involvement with their participants that stems from the subjective nature of qualitative research. As highlighted in Chapter 3, qualitative researchers must initiate a rapport-building process from their first encounter with a participant in order to build a research relationship that will allow the researcher access to that person's story (Ceglowski, 2000;

Goodwin *et al.*, 2003; Grbich, 2007; Liamputtong & Ezzy, 2005; Minichiello *et al.*, 2000; Payne, 1994; Taylor & Bogdan, 1998). The rapport-building process may introduce a situation that contributes to a merging of boundaries between researcher and participant. For example, some of the rapport-building strategies used by the researchers we interviewed included such things as sharing a meal, attending family gatherings, looking at family photos and running errands. As part of this process the researcher utilizes self-examination, sharing and self-disclosure to develop rapport and trust (Campbell & Wasco, 2000; Oakley, 1981; Stanley & Wise, 1991). Steven Taylor and Robert Bogdan (1998:48) highlight that in order to enter people's lives for the purposes of research, researchers need to communicate 'a feeling of empathy for informants', 'penetrate people's defences' and have 'people open up about their feelings'. The ability to do this is important in all qualitative research, but particularly so for sensitive research, as people may be asked to talk about intimate aspects of their lives. Some of the researchers interviewed spoke about the importance of being professional.

Sometimes it is important to remind yourself that you are a professional researcher – that you are doing research – that you are not their counsellor that you are not some kind of service provider – that you are listening to their story and that's all you are doing.

I am not the same person when I am doing interviews with people. I do things differently when I am interviewing, I am a professional and I have to act like one.

Some of the researchers interviewed intentionally initiated the self-protection strategy of staying somehow detached from the research, so that they did not end up crossing those boundaries.

In a sense I needed to remain outside to protect myself from the research.

I tried to remove myself from what she was telling me. Trying hard not to think about aspects of my own childhood that were similar to hers. I wanted to be a professional and not get wrapped up in the story.

I am able to mentally detach from the situation, I do this to stay outside the research.

However, this strategy did not work for all researchers and many of the researchers that were interviewed spoke about the difficulties they faced in managing the boundaries particularly when they began sharing their own stories throughout the research process. When researchers become involved in this type of reciprocal sharing the maintenance of professional detachment becomes extremely difficult.

Despite the fact that researcher self-disclosure is often cited as good research practice (see the discussion in Chapter 3), particularly in feminist research (Oakley, 1981; Reinharz, 1992), clinicians have been warned against undertaking any level of self-disclosure to their clients as it may 'open the door to boundary problems' (Walker & Clark, 1999:1438). The counselling literature highlights many of the negative aspects of boundary blurring, focusing particularly on exploitation of clients (Corey, Corey & Callanan, 2003; Hart & Wright-Crawford, 1999; Hartmann, 1997; Hermansson, 1997; Petronio, 1991). This exploitation can be described more generally as a 'boundary violation' defined by Arnold Lazarus and Ofer Zur (2002:6) as 'actions on the part of the clinician that are harmful, exploitative'. In contrast to this, boundary crossing has also been described as a more benign means of enhancing relationships between clients and professionals (Scopelliti *et al.*, 2004). Researchers, like clinicians, need to think through how much self-disclosure they will undertake in the process of the research.

Boundaries between friendship and research

Researchers often talk about developing friendships with the people whom they research (Acker *et al.*, 1991; Cannon, 1992; Gair, 2002; Johnson & Clarke, 2003; Liamputtong Rice, 2000; Stebbins, 1991; Watson, Irwin & Michalske, 1991). As observed by Raymond Lee (1993:107), researchers often become involved in a 'growing closeness, which creates a blurred line between the role of friend and that of research participant'. One of the researchers we interviewed stated:

With a lot of them it did become like a friendship, we shared something that at times was quite intimate . . . they had told me stories about their lives, including their sexual lives, and that sort of takes the research relationship beyond a certain level.

Lynne Watson, Jeanette Irwin and Sharon Michalske (1991:509), use the term 'researcher-friend', recognizing that researchers often get involved in friendship-like relationships with research participants. Sue Cannon (1989:66) spoke of going through a 'transition to friendship' with her participants that included having cups of tea, sometimes joining them for meals and giving small gifts to her and her children. Others spoke about meeting partners and children (Acker *et al.*, 1991) and undertaking small friendship gestures like giving small gifts and sending Christmas cards (Liamputtong Rice, 2000; Watson *et al.*, 1991).

Qualitative researchers spend a considerable amount of time in participants' homes, often staying with a participant after an interview to share a cup of tea or take a walk in the garden. For researchers working in sensitive areas, the difficulties in managing the boundaries are often heightened due to the amount of time and energy spent in developing rapport and trust. It has also been said that researchers may fake friendships (Duncombe & Jessop, 2002) in order to gain their data. As previously highlighted, although these courtesies are important for rapport maintenance they may also create an expectation that the research relationship becomes more like a friendship. One of the researchers interviewed comments:

I sometimes feel like perhaps just on the littlest level that they might feel that you are a friend and you feel a teeny bit guilty cause they are giving you cups of tea and being really nice.

For some of those we interviewed, the relationship with participants moved beyond that of an interviewer/interviewee and became more about having someone to talk to. In one instance, a researcher, who had carried out a number of interviews with each research participant, described how the relationship she had with one woman changed.

By the time I got to the last interview, she said 'I don't want to talk about this anymore I'm over it, I want to talk about the garden, talk about my family, talk about this and that' and it was almost like – me being the researcher, I wasn't there as a researcher, I was there as a friend. Like in terms of, 'okay, we've talked about this to death and I'm sick of it and I've got nothing else to offer you but I still really like you being here and because we have gotten on so well I am happy for you to be here but I just don't want to talk about what you want to talk about'.

Instead of being there in a research capacity, this researcher felt that she was now going into the woman's home in the role of a friend. This raises a number of issues for researchers who obviously cannot continue visiting participants indefinitely but also feel some obligation to continue relationships with participants because they have often shared so much of themselves in the telling of their stories.

Sometimes the development of friendships reflected the fact that some of the people who participate in research appear to need someone to be their friend. As stated earlier, many of the researchers who were interviewed undertook research with marginalized and vulnerable people who may have been particularly 'needy'. Often researchers felt that they could offer some level of friendship but many were clear that it would not be able to be an ongoing friendship.

I struggled about it – they were lonely people and they wanted a friend and I didn't really want to offer that . . . not in an ongoing way.

One researcher told of inviting a research participant over to share Christmas dinner, which was traditionally a family event, because the participant had been so helpful in the research.

She was just – she was kinda smart and good and she had these nice little kids and you know – it was kind of a bit of kindness but also she was a pretty nice woman, she'd been really helpful and it really was the least I could do.

Others we interviewed spoke about sharing a range of social occasions with participants, acknowledging that sometimes it just feels right to be involved in people's lives to that extent, especially when you have been with that person over a difficult or extended period of time. Many of the researchers who spoke about developing friendships with participants attributed it to the fact that the friendships developed as a natural progression due to the nature of what the researcher and the participant were sharing.

I mean I would be friendly and there is this woman whose husband died last year and she invited me around a couple of times for a meal and then the last time I took my husband and made it more of a social thing and she really enjoyed that. I am open to doing this like that if it seems like a good thing at the time. I mean I was with her through a lot of difficult things.

Others reported the difficulties of maintaining friendships with research participants, often feeling quite overwhelmed by the expectations.

Like I got 35 new friends and I'd only had probably maybe two or three mates in my entire life you know and I had these guys, these 35 relationships with these guys and now some of them took that further you know – like I went up to Brisbane [4000 km away] and stayed a week with one of the guys and his wife. I felt like I owed them that much after what they had given to me.

As previously discussed, some researchers do develop relationships with the participants that border on friendship and this can make leaving the field and ending the relationship problematic. Some of the researchers wondered how they were going to feel when the research was over, referring specifically to the difficulties they were expecting to face ending the relationship with the participants.

It is really hard to imagine how I am going to end this. I have come to know these people, you know sometimes I drop by and have a cup of tea, sit and talk, have a look at the photos from the latest holiday.

For some researchers the realization that they will not be able to continue friendships with those involved in their research comes to the fore when the participant dies. Given the nature of the topics that the researchers undertaking sensitive research might be investigating (for example HIV, cancer, death or other areas that involved interviewing people who had life-threatening illnesses) this is not a rare or entirely unexpected occurrence. However, this may add to the difficulties associated with developing friendships.

I really liked her and I went back on a number of occasions and she then passed away and it was then when I really started thinking more clearly about the boundaries and realizing that if I continued to do qualitative research there was no way that I could keep up friends with all those people.

The ongoing nature of the relationship is something that takes some researchers by surprise and they often do not have strategies in place to deal with that.

At the very beginning of this research study we thought we had worked everything out, all the things that might happen during the data collection, but we had not factored in becoming friends with these people and how we would deal with that.

Some researchers do maintain a level of contact with participants in their research studies, sometimes over an extended period of time following completion of the study. Researchers use different methods to stay in touch including writing letters, emails, phone calls, maintaining some social contact and sending Christmas cards (Hubbard *et al.*, 2001; Robertson, 2000; Watson *et al.*, 1991). The amount of contact differs considerably, from some having minimal contact to those who had extended contact for a number of years post completion.

I have been in contact with those people for eight years now, on and off. Once a year or thereabouts I correspond with them and I continue to send Christmas cards to everyone who was in my doctoral research.

It's not like I maintain contact with them on a regular basis, but I do still send them cards at Christmas time and they often send them back to me as well. I don't know how long I'll keep doing that, I guess it will end one day.

While sending Christmas greetings to research participants may be a popular way of maintaining contact, there may be some difficulties associated with this.

I talked to my supervisor about saying goodbye to them and she said 'why don't you send them Christmas cards?', but the thing is – I mean with cancer research you don't know do you? They could be dead and then the family is going to get it and they might not even know that she was in the research. You can't ever tell. I rang someone this morning to organize another interview and she was fine six months ago but now she is palliative – I don't think she'll be around for Christmas.

Leaving the field can be difficult in any research situation, particularly for researchers of sensitive topics (Cannon, 1989; Hubbard *et al.*, 2001; Russell, 1999; Stebbins, 1991; Warren, 2002), which has led Robert Stebbins (1991:253) to pose the question 'Do we ever leave the field?' Issues around 'leaving the field' are not new and were also raised by Sue Cannon (1989:74) who reported difficulties in leaving the field in her study of breast cancer. She felt from the outset that it would be very difficult to ever completely leave the field. In her study of breast cancer, 21 women died and she talks of being affected by all of the deaths. She noted that she felt a number of emotions including sadness, depression, shock, anger and feelings of great loss.

Gayle Burr (1995:174) has named the difficulty associated with leaving the field as 'unfinished business' and highlights that researchers can experience 'on-going feelings of concern for the fate of each person' (1995:177). As Carol Warren (2002:96) states, 'like most things, qualitative interviews come to an end [. . .] but sometimes [. . .] Interviewers do not necessarily end their relationship with respondents at the conclusion of their interview'. Researchers have articulated a concern that sometimes it feels like research participants are 'living inside their heads' (Goodrum & Keys, 2007; Kleinman & Copp, 1993; Warr, 2004). Other difficulties documented in leaving the field may indicate that researchers are both physically and emotionally immersed in the research (Atkinson, Coffey & Delamont, 2003; Cannon, 1992) and although our relationships with research participants may only be short term, this 'does not prevent their ending from signifying a loss' (Atkinson *et al.*, 2003:55). The ending of a research interview does not always signify an ending of thoughts about the research participants and it is important that researchers think through the process of disengaging from the field.

Research or counselling/therapy and the 'quasitherapeutic' relationship

The therapeutic nature of participation in research has been raised repeatedly (Birch & Miller, 2000; Burr, 1995; Gale, 1992; Higgins, 1998; Rosenblatt, 1995; Rowling, 1999; Sque, 2000). While it is important for researchers not to underestimate the therapeutic value of participating in research on some sensitive topics, it is also important for researchers to be aware of the fact that people may be offering to participate hoping for therapeutic outcomes, rather than simply a desire to tell their story.

Concerns about the therapeutic role of research interviews have been raised (Coyle, 1998; Etherington, 1996; Grafanaki, 1996; King, 1996; Mauthner, Birch, Jessop & Miller, 2002) and some of the parallels between research and therapy interviews have been documented. Some aspects of research interviews are strikingly similar to aspects of therapeutic interviews (see Box 4.1).

Many of the researchers we interviewed reported that the participants in their studies found participation to be of therapeutic benefit.

It's not like I had done anything except provide them a space to talk, and that's what therapy is . . . part of what therapy is anyway.

I do believe that the process of telling and having an empathetic listener who is prepared to spend the time with that person is therapeutic in itself.

Box 4.1 Similarities between therapeutic interviews and qualitative research interviews

- both provide a space to talk
- empathetic listening
- uninterrupted opportunity to share a personal story
- seek to empower the participant
- intense interviewing sessions where one person often divulges personal information to another person whose role it is to listen and ask questions.

Both research and therapeutic interviews provide a space for people to talk about their experiences to someone who really wants to listen (Duncombe & Jessop, 2002; Hutchinson & Wilson, 1994). As highlighted by Jean Duncombe and Julie Jessop (2002:112), 'even skilled researchers may find it difficult to draw neat boundaries around 'rapport', 'friendship' and 'intimacy', in order to avoid the depths of 'counselling' and 'therapy''. Another similarity between research and therapy/counselling interviews is that they both seek to empower the people who choose to take part. Both involve intense interviewing sessions, where one person often divulges personal information to another person whose role it is to listen and ask questions.

One of the reasons for the difficulties faced by researchers in managing the boundaries between research and counselling/therapy is that they both require similar skills (Coyle & Wright, 1996; Glesne & Peshkin, 1992; Hutchinson & Wilson, 1994; Kvale, 1996). For example, empathy and listening skills are emphasized as being important for both research interviews (particularly qualitative interviews on sensitive topics) and for counselling or therapy interviews (Corey *et al.*, 2003; Glesne & Peshkin, 1992; Kvale, 1996; Liamputtong Rice & Ezzy, 1999; Minichiello *et al.*, 2000; Renzetti & Lee, 1993; Walker & Clark, 1999). Some research interviews can take hours to complete and research relationships can last for a number of years. This kind of intense contact often surpasses the amount of contact that people have throughout a therapeutic process and in some instances participants may find qualitative research interviews to be of more therapeutic value than therapy interviews (Gale, 1992).

In order to somehow draw a line between research and therapy one researcher expressed how she differentiated one from the other:

I don't think I'm doing therapy as such, I'm not actually offering people an ongoing relationship but I think there are certain aspects that could be linked to therapy and I'm not sure if the people who take part know the difference.

The difficulties associated with characterizing therapy as requiring an ongoing relationship are that many researchers *do* end up developing some kind of longer term relationships with their participants (see the earlier discussion around research and friendship and consider an example of qualitative research that consists of regular interviews over a number of months or years).

Research participants have reported participating in qualitative research as both enjoyable and personally rewarding (Cook & Bosley, 1995; Hutchinson *et al.*, 1994; Kondora, 1993; Liamputtong Rice, 2000). Participants have felt relief and a sense of catharsis from the sharing of their stories (Brannen, 1988, 1993; Cowles, 1988; Lee & Renzetti, 1993; Murray, 2003; Owens, 1996; Platzer & James, 1997; Sque, 2000). Claire Draucker (1999:164) reports that her participants felt that 'their participation was beneficial to them, usually because it gave them an opportunity to share their thoughts and feelings and possibly help other victims of violence'. So, while some participants may take part in research for altruistic reasons, the participants themselves may also gain from their participation.

Some of the researchers we interviewed raised concerns about their role in the research and reported a sense of unease about the therapeutic value of their research. There appeared to be a sense of confusion about whether researchers should, or indeed could, avoid being placed in a therapeutic role by those they interviewed.

I think they [research participants] find it very therapeutic, especially if it's something that they haven't talked about before. They're in a situation where they are actually being invited to talk about it and that in itself acknowledges that it's an issue that's worth talking about and that's important.

I found that time and time again, at the end of the interview people said, 'oh thank you, thank you so much, I never get a chance to talk about this, I've never talked about that to anyone, it was really great, your questions were fantastic and they really gave me a chance to talk about it in the open . . . it's over now'.

Some of the researchers that we interviewed spoke about the conflict they encountered in the conduct of research because of their other professional roles. Many of them had undergone professional training or had previous professional backgrounds, some of which included counselling, therapy, social work, nursing, advocacy and teaching. Many of those with dual roles or training spoke about the difficulty in maintaining the professional boundaries between those roles. These issues have also been previously raised in the literature (Etherington, 1996; Lalor *et al.*, 2006; Richards & Schwartz, 2002). When researchers are directly involved in the care of the participant, the interview process is more likely to be confused with a therapeutic encounter and this may lead them to disclose more information than they had antici-pated when consenting to participate in the study (Richards & Schwartz, 2002). The researchers interviewed who identified role conflict as an issue spoke of the importance of ensuring that the participants were clear that the researcher was not providing therapy, but conducting an interview to collect information. Some researchers may feel an urge to adopt a position of a proxy counsellor or therapist to research participants who are in distress (Bloor, Fincham & Sampson, 2007) as it is very difficult to spend time with someone who is obviously distressed and not offer anything (Allan, 2006; Copp, 1998; Dickson-Swift, James, Kippen *et al.*, 2006; Johnson & Clarke, 2003; Kvale, 1996).

Some of the researchers we interviewed did have counselling experience and some felt that these skills helped them to deal effectively with some of the issues raised in research on sensitive topics. However, others felt that the possession of counselling or therapy skills only complicated the process and made it more difficult for the researcher to delineate between the role of the researcher and the role of the counsellor.

So, while there are many similarities between therapy and research interviews there are also some important differences. In a therapy interview, the therapist is listening to the participant and helping that person, whereas in the latter, the participant is helping the researcher by providing information (Birch & Miller, 2000; Hart & Wright-Crawford, 1999). Conversely, the participant may also be helped if the process of telling another person is therapeutic in itself. This point has been raised by Hutchinson and Wilson (1994:305) who seek to remind researchers that their 'major role is that of scientist'. While it would be difficult to disagree with this, qualitative researchers involved in research on sensitive topics are often listening to people talk about highly personal aspects of their lives, which may involve raising some unresolved and/or emotional issues. In this case, it is possible that participation in a research interview has some therapeutic pay-offs for the participant.

In support of this, some feminist writers have considered the possibility that there may be some therapeutic pay-offs or opportunities for personal growth afforded to those who participate in research interviews, stating that this may be more evident in research interviews where people are encouraged to talk about themselves and to examine in-depth parts of their lives (Bergen, 1993; Brannen, 1993). These therapeutic pay-offs may be extended to the researcher as well as the participant. Participation in research has the potential to transform both participants and researchers (Ellis *et al.*, 1997; Kiesinger, 1998; Kleinman, 1991; Rosenblatt, 2001).

Researchers may consciously avoid getting involved in a therapy session; a qualitative researcher's ability to listen may lead to what has been termed a 'quasitherapeutic' relationship (Kvale, 1996:155). One of the main problems with this is that if the participant finds the interviews therapeutic it may lead them to talk about deeper personal problems that in turn require therapeutic assistance. Most researchers do not have appropriate training in therapeutic support to deal with such situations. Concern has been raised over researchers finding themselves in the role of a therapist without any appropriate training or experience in therapy (Hart & Wright-Crawford, 1999). When there is an overlap between the roles of researcher and therapist there is the potential for some ethical issues to arise that have not been fully addressed prior to undertaking the research. One of the issues may be that the researcher needs to consider what he/she is consenting to when a research relationship is established with a participant, and how the boundaries should be managed from the researcher's perspective (Miller & Boulton, 2007).

Offering participant debriefing and referrals is often cited as good qualitative research practice (Grbich, 1999; Ribbens & Edwards, 1998; Tee & Lathlean, 2004). Providing support mechanisms and debriefing have also been indicated as being helpful for researchers working on sensitive issues (Tee & Lathlean, 2004). Alty and Rodham (1998:208) suggest that 'researchers embarking on a project that focuses on sensitive issues would not be fulfilling their obligations to respondents if they did not 'debrief' the respondents and talk through the complex issues and feelings they may have aroused'. Although we may agree with this idea in theory, the reality is that many researchers do not feel adequately trained to participate in that level of debriefing and may in fact do more harm than good.

I'm not a counsellor – you know I'm not a therapist, I'm not a social worker – I'm a sociologist – and I am an amateur bumbling around in peoples lives if I try and do something that I am not trained at – so if I try and get in there and fix some of this stuff I am incredibly likely to make a big bloody mess of it!

So, while some participants may be helped by telling their story there is the possibility that others may be left requiring some therapeutic assistance. Researchers often arm themselves with referral mechanisms, tissues and pamphlets in case participants need some help, and they are often left feeling a little unclear about their role.

I dunno how I felt about that, she opened up and told me her story in all its sordid detail, she was not good, and really neither was I. I dunno sometimes I feel like I am not the right person to do this – like I'm not qualified to do this for these people. It felt so superficial when I said, 'here are some numbers and some pamphlets – perhaps you need to talk to someone'.

. . . so we sort of stopped and talked about it for a minute in terms of getting help but that's all I can do – I can't physically take her somewhere and I can't say – 'how do you feel about that?', you know I can't – I'm not there to offer that sort of role.

On the whole, researchers are not required to be trained therapists or counsellors, and if they allow the research to turn into therapy they may not be able to handle the situations that may arise. When the interview is conceptualized as having both research and therapeutic merit it may lead to difficulties for both researchers and participants (Hewitt, 2007). However, despite the fact that many researchers are not trained counsellors or therapists it is possible that participants will find the exercise therapeutic. This could be a source of stress and confusion for researchers who may feel that they do not have the necessary skills or training to administer therapy.

I think it is a form of therapy and I'm not quite sure how comfortable I feel about that because I am not a trained therapist, or a counsellor and I try very hard not to do that.

It's really hard, particularly as a researcher, you are not there to help them, you are there to collect data and I find it quite impersonal, but at the same time I'm not equipped to counsel, I'm not equipped to really deal with issues.

Some of the researchers we interviewed raised concerns that in the process of the research interview they were often asking people to retell their stories and that this may initiate an opening up of old wounds or an exploration of previously hidden information.

I worry about this cause they haven't gone into it and perhaps there are certain reasons why they haven't gone into it before and then I ask them to talk about it and that's really leaving someone open, open to all sorts of things.

One important aspect of the discussion regarding issues of therapy and research is that while research interviews may have a therapeutic value for participants, researchers acknowledge that this therapeutic value was completely unintentional. Corrine Glense and Alan Peshkin (1992:123) have also recognized this dilemma, attesting that, 'although researchers do not wittingly assume the role of therapist, they nonetheless fashion an interview process that can be strikingly therapeutic'.

I didn't set out for this to happen but overwhelmingly people commented on the value that this process was to them.

. . . so whilst I know that researchers can't be therapists for all kinds of good, practical, theoretical, ethical reasons you can't avoid the fact that your intervention in that person's life has an effect on that person and we must take that responsibility seriously.

Tina Miller (2007:2208), notes that one of her participants in research with fathers explicitly told her via email that the 'interviews have been a little like counselling. I think we can all do with a little gentle counselling'. Whether or not researchers are adequately prepared for this role is contentious.

Potential implications of poor boundary management

As highlighted at the beginning of this chapter, researchers may be concerned about their roles in sensitive research, sometimes feeling more like a counsellor than a researcher, or more like a friend than a researcher, or unprofessional when they react emotionally during an interview. This ambiguity of roles for professionals is frequently cited as a source of occupational stress (Beehr, 1995; Dollard, 2003; Kay, 2000). Researchers (like other professionals) need to be clear about their role in the research process. Concerns over roles, maintaining professional distance, and being detached but concerned, all add additional stress to research work (Johnson & Clarke, 2003; Johnson & Plant, 1996). If the call from some feminist researchers to blur the distinction between researchers and researched is heeded (Acker *et al.*, 1991; Hertz, 1997), it is imperative that researchers are equipped with the skills to deal with the additional stress this may introduce.

As we discussed in Chapter 3, emotional exhaustion and feeling overwhelmed has been identified as one of the main threats to researchers in sensitive research (Cannon, 1992; McCosker *et al.*, 2001; Parker & Ulrich, 1990). Heather McCosker and her colleagues (2001:4) reported that 'the sense of emotional exhaustion and being overwhelmed by the nature of the interviewee's experience can be extreme'. This sense of emotional exhaustion,

Table 4.1. Consequences of burn-out

Thematic category	Specific consequences
Mental consequences	Lowered self-esteem
	Depression
	Irritability
	Helplessness
	Anxiety
	Diminished frustration tolerance
	Cognitive impairment
Physical consequences	Fatigue
	Insomnia
	Headaches
	Gastrointestinal disturbances
	Sexual problems
	Increased incidence of illness
	Increased risk of cardiovascular disease
Behavioural consequences	Personal neglect – poor diet and reduced physical activity
	Aggression
	Increased use of caffeine and other substances
Attitudinal consequences	Negative attitudes towards clients or job, organization and self
Social consequences	Withdrawal from social contact
	Decreased involvement with recipients
	Negative spill over from work to home

(*Source:* derived from Griffiths, 2003:373)

leaving their research encounters feeling emotionally drained, has also been reported by other writers (Dunn, 1991; Goodrum & Keys, 2007; Moran-Ellis, 1996; Stanko, 1997).

Researchers who feel overwhelmed and emotionally exhausted may be at risk of burn-out. Although the experience of burn-out has been well documented among health professionals, the concept of researcher burn-out is underdeveloped. Individuals in many of the 'people work' occupations report that over time they can become emotionally exhausted (Maslach, 1982; Pennebaker, 1990). Professions with the highest rates of burn-out in the health professions include nursing and social work (Cherniss, 1995). Susan Griffiths (2003:371) has summarized the correlates of burn-out, showing the variables and the direction of their effects from a number of studies examining occupational stress in the service professions. In Table 4.1 we have summarized the main consequences of burn-out.

As many of the reported studies are cross-sectional in design no causality can be inferred; however, it is interesting to note that positive correlations between role conflict, role ambiguity and boundary management were identified. Griffiths' (2003:373) table of the consequences of burn-out (see Table 4.1) also documents many of the physical problems reported as specific consequences of burn-out, including anxiety, fatigue, insomnia, headaches and gastrointestinal disturbances, which are similar to symptoms reported by researchers working in sensitive research have reported. A number of writers have stated that researchers may be negatively emotionally and physically affected by research on sensitive issues (Alexander *et al.*, 1989; Burr, 1995; Cowles, 1988; Dunn, 1991; Gregory *et al.*, 1997; Lee, 1995; McCosker *et al.*, 2001). Some of the possible negative outcomes include gastrointestinal problems (Dunn, 1991), insomnia and nightmares (Cowles, 1988; Dunn, 1991; Etherington, 1996), headaches (Dunn, 1991), exhaustion and depression (Ridge *et al.*, 1999). It is well documented that undertaking sensitive research can be a distressing experience (Campbell, 2002; Cannon, 1992; Dunn, 1991; Gair, 2002; Rowling, 1999) that can leave researchers feeling emotionally and physically drained.

Emotional distancing has been cited as a useful measure to address occupational stress in human service occupations. This distancing can enable professionals to actively manage the boundaries between themselves and their clients and is a well accepted strategy used by social workers (Bennett *et al.*, 1993; Lonne, 2003). While there may be some value in researchers using emotional distancing as a strategy to manage burn-out the skills involved are not routinely covered in research training.

Professionals in many health disciplines have codes of practice that govern their everyday work practices. Many of these professional codes (see for example, Australian Association of Social Workers, 1999; Australian Guidance and Counselling Association, 1997; Australian Psychological Society, 2002) include the provision of formalized support and debriefing for the workers as standard practice. This type of support acts not only as a check upon clinical practice but also as a safeguard for both the client and the professional (Brannen, 1988). Many researchers do not have the same level of formalized support that is available to other professionals dealing with sensitive situations. Julia Brannen (1988:562) speaks of her experience, 'having sat sometimes for several hours at a time in people's homes listening to their stories and to their distress I have often thought that no psychiatrist or psychotherapist would work (or be allowed to work) under these conditions'. The provision of support and the opportunity for debriefing may act as a protective mechanism to help ensure that researchers are not adversely affected by the work that they do. The important role that debriefing may play in protecting researchers from psychological harm is discussed further in Chapter 7.

The issues surrounding the identification and management of boundaries between clients and professionals has also been recognized by many professional bodies and are embedded in professional ethical codes (see for example in Australia, Australian Association of Social Workers, 1999; Australian Guidance and Counselling Association, 1997; Australian Nursing Council, 2003; Australian Psychological Society, 2002; Nurses Board of Victoria, 2001). Most of these codes have explicit guidelines for professionals about the management of relationships and the setting and maintenance of professional boundaries. Researchers are answerable to institutional ethics committees (IECs), but these do not currently identify boundary issues, as discussed here and documented in the literature, as coming within their frame of reference (Dickson-Swift, James & Kippen, 2005).

Despite the fact that qualitative researchers face a number of challenges in managing boundaries when undertaking research, comprehensive recommendations for researchers and research supervisors are lacking. Given the implications of poor boundary management, researchers, research supervisors and IECs involved in this type of research are urged to consider protocols in the following areas outlined in Box 4.2.

The difficulties for researchers in this situation are similar to those experienced by counsellors. As Gary Hermansson (1997:143) states, 'it is especially important for counsellors to be able to understand and monitor their own processes, personally and through ongoing supervision, and to recognise signs of burn-out as this is often where boundary-management process problems begin'. This advice could well be taken up by researchers, enabling them to better manage the boundaries in sensitive research, benefiting both themselves and their participants. Research supervisors might use these issues as a basis for discussions with less experienced researchers to help them to plan self-protection strategies. It is envisaged that if researchers and research supervisors give consideration to each of these areas they will be better placed to manage the many different boundaries issues inherent in qualitative research.

We recommended that researchers and research supervisors involved in qualitative research on sensitive topics explore the boundaries that may arise in their research and have in place some strategies to deal with any 'blurring' that may occur. We also recommended training be provided to assist

---

Box 4.2 Suggested areas for protocol development

- disclosure
- rapport
- clarity around therapy versus research
- strategies for leaving the research relationship
- the management of professional boundaries including friendships.

researchers to recognize and manage any boundary issues that may arise. Such training would provide researchers with the skills to effectively manage some of the boundaries identified and ensure that researchers are not adversely affected by their participation in research.

Summary

How then do researchers maintain responsible boundaries in research while incorporating some boundary crossing with participants in order to develop the empathy and rapport needed to undertake the research? Boundary issues surrounding the professional conduct of qualitative research including the development of rapport, use of researcher self-disclosure and need for support have been examined in this chapter. The difficulties associated with differentiating between research interviews and a therapy/counselling situation have been presented, and problems associated with maintaining boundaries between friendship and research have been explored. A number of potential serious and negative consequences for researchers who do not manage the boundaries in research have been highlighted. These include difficulties in leaving research relationships, researchers feeling emotionally and physically overwhelmed by the commitments placed upon them, physical symptoms and risk of burn-out. While this chapter reflects the experiences of the researchers interviewed who were all involved in sensitive research, the possibility that other researchers may face similar issues with boundary blurring cannot be discounted.

Tutorial activities

(a) One of the boundaries that many researchers report difficulty in establishing and sustaining is the boundary between researcher and therapist. Reflect on your own personal skills in conducting therapeutic interviews. What will you do if a participant asks for your advice about what they should do? How will you proceed? What advice will you give them? What strategies can you put in place to help ensure that the research interview does not become seen as a therapeutic opportunity for the participant?

(b) Another important boundary is that between researcher and friend. Consider the following scenario. You are conducting a series of interviews with cancer patients exploring the impact of a cancer diagnosis on their family and social relationships. You are going to be interviewing the participants in their homes over a period of months and development of rapport will be very important. What strategies will you use to disengage from the research relationship when the study is over?

SUGGESTED READING

Birch, M. & Miller, T. (2000). Inviting intimacy: the interview as therapeutic opportunity. *International Journal of Social Research Methodology*, **3**(3), 189–202.

Dickson-Swift, V., James, E., Kippen, S. & Liamputtong, P. (2006a). Blurring boundaries in qualitative health research on sensitive topics. *Qualitative Health Research*, **16**(6), 853–871.

Etherington, K. (1996). The counsellor as researcher: boundary issues and critical dilemmas. *British Journal of Guidance and Counselling*, **24**(3), 339–346.

Hart, N. & Wright-Crawford, N. (1999). Research as therapy, therapy as research: ethical dilemmas in new-paradigm research. *British Journal of Guidance and Counselling*, **27**(2), 205–214.

Hermansson, G. (1997). Boundaries and boundary management in counselling: the never-ending story. *British Journal of Guidance and Counselling*, **25**(2), 133–145.

Walker, R. & Clark, J. (1999). Heading off boundary problems: clinical supervision as risk management. *Psychiatric Services*, **50**(11), 1435–1439.

5

Emotions and sensitive research

It has become increasingly fashionable for individual researchers to 'personalise' their accounts of fieldwork. But there has been little systematic attempt to reflect upon their experiences and emotions that are reported in any overarching collective or epistemological sense.

(Coffey, 1999:1)

There is a growing awareness that undertaking qualitative research on sensitive topics is an embodied experience and that researchers may be emotionally affected by the work that they do; however, empirical attention to the emotional nature of research is lacking. In this chapter we provide a number of different conceptualizations of emotions and examine their relevance for research work on sensitive topics. In order to understand the emotional nature of qualitative research on sensitive topics we also examine the sociological literature pertinent to emotion work and explore how the theories of emotional labour and emotion work can be applied to the experience of undertaking sensitive research.

As we have outlined in earlier chapters, undertaking qualitative research on sensitive topics requires interaction with people in order to understand and document their experiences. To do this we need to acknowledge that 'Qualitative social research is 'people work' and is therefore also 'emotional work'' (Lee-Treweek, 2000:128). Liz Stoler (2002:270) reminds us that 'emotional reactions and personal needs do not just vanish because one has declared oneself a researcher'. Acknowledging and documenting the emotion work required from researchers to do this type of research may help us to understand some of the difficulties they face.

Defining emotions

Emotion has been defined as a sensuous, cognitive and social/cultural experience (Burkitt, 1997; Lupton, 1998). Defining emotion is very difficult as the term 'emotion' is used to describe a wide range of different things (Jaggar, 1989). Liz Stanley and Sue Wise (1983) claim that *emotions* are products of the mind and are different from *feelings*, which are responses of the body. For example, Alison Jaggar (1989) highlights that cold and pain are *feelings* whereas love and envy are *emotions*. Describing emotion in this way is quite simplistic and disembodied as it asserts that the mind and the body experience emotion in different ways. This ideal has been termed *Cartesian dualism*, focusing on the separation of mind and body and seeing them as separate entities (Turner, 1992). Alison Jaggar (1989) elaborates on this idea by suggesting that feelings can be linked to physiological sensations while emotions include some conscious aspects as well as the physiological ones. This theory has been extended and now encompasses the idea that emotion can be linked to physiological sensations. Therefore, if feeling an emotion has aspects of cognitive and physiological sensations it can be said that we can feel as well as think (Hochschild, 1979; Jaggar, 1989).

Simon Williams (1998:750) further developed the definition of emotion, stating that, 'emotions, in other words are *emergent* properties, located at the intersection of physiological *dispositions*, material *circumstances* and sociocultural *elaboration*' (his emphasis). Arlie Hochschild (1990:118–119) sees emotion as an awareness of four elements experienced at the same time: (a) appraisal of a situation, (b) changes in bodily sensations, (c) the freeing of inhibited display of expressive gestures, and (d) a cultural label applied to specific constellations of the first three elements. She goes on to state that a feeling is also an emotion but it has a much less marked bodily sensation. It is therefore, a milder emotion. Peggy Thoits (1990:191) presents the constituents of emotion as four interconnected components: (a) situational cues, (b) physiological changes, (c) expressive gestures, and (d) an emotion label that identifies these components. Similarly, June Crawford and colleagues (1992) define emotion as involving affect or feelings and cognition, stating that they are expressions of inner feelings that communicate our feelings to other people. One important feature of all the authors' definitions is an agreement that when we feel an emotion we must somehow communicate it to ourselves. This processing of information to the self has been said to possess a 'signal function' (Hochschild, 1990), alerting us that an emotion is being felt.

Emotion is a fundamental part of human life and one aspect of our humanness is our capacity to feel and to show emotion (Gilbert, 2001a). As Norman Denzin (1984:x) illustrates:

emotionality lies at the intersection of the person and society, for all persons are joined to their societies through the self-feelings and emotions they feel and experience on a daily basis. This is the reason the study of emotionality must occupy a central place in all the human disciplines, for to be human is to be emotional.

If emotionality does lie at the intersection of the person and society then it follows that emotions are a central part of the research process. As qualitative researchers, our goal is to see the world through someone else's eyes, using ourselves as a research instrument; it thus follows that we must experience our research 'both intellectually and emotionally' (Gilbert, 2001a:9). As researchers, we should see research not only as an intellectual exercise but also 'as a process of exploration and discovery that is felt deeply' (Gilbert, 2001a:9). Researchers have defined emotions to be 'feelings, sensations, drives; the personal; that which is intimate; personally meaningful, possibly overwhelming; being touched at a deeper level; something that comes from somewhere within ourselves; and that which makes us truly human' (Gilbert, 2001a:9).

Understanding how emotions are entwined in the research process can be linked to ontological and epistemological views. How do we come to know what we know and who can know? Under a positivist framework, which strongly advocates for an objectivist stance of reality that can be measured and verified, emotions can be seen as an unnecessary source of bias. Positivist science would have us believe that we, as researchers, must find ways to minimize these types of potential bias. Some of the later postpositivist theorists like Jürgen Habermas (1971, 1988) began to question the existence of an objective reality and postulated that instead 'reality' is socially constructed. Undertaking research is a subjective experience, especially undertaking qualitative research, whereby the researcher interacts with the participants in order to collect the data. To do this type of research, we, as researchers, need to make use of our humanness in the research. This humanness comprises being open to our emotions and acknowledging the role that emotions play in research.

While researchers firmly entrenched in the scientific paradigm may not feel able to speak about their emotions in their research, researchers working from the interpretive paradigm may be more able to do so. In this paradigm, the role of the subjective experience in the research process is valued (Denzin & Lincoln, 1994). While this shift to the interpretive paradigm and its subsequent acceptance of the subjective nature of research has allowed for the researcher to be considered in the research, feminist methodology provided some of the impetus for the examination of the role of researcher's emotion in the research process (Jaggar, 1989; Stanley, 1990; Stanley & Wise, 1983). As outlined in Chapter 2, feminist researchers have long argued for researchers to acknowledge their own feelings as part of the research process, taking into account the values of reflexivity and reciprocity (Stanley & Wise, 1983, 1993). In contrast, one of the main criticisms of emotions in research has been articulated by Carolyn Ellis (1991) who asserts that often emotion has come to be viewed by some as a type of over-rapport leading to a fear from some researchers of what has been termed 'going native' (Van Maanen,

1990a) and becoming too heavily involved in the research. It is important for researchers to acknowledge their feelings as part of the research process by taking into account both the 'thinking' and the 'feeling' aspects of the research (Campbell, 2002).

Emotions in research

Academic interest in emotion has been gathering momentum since the 1970s. For example, social researchers like Colin Bell and Howard Newby (1977) and Bell and Saul Encel (1978) drew attention to the importance of writing accounts of the difficulties researchers face in fieldwork and that it is necessary for the researchers to place themselves in the research. William Shaffir, Robert Stebbins and Allan Turowetz (1980:3–4) make this point:

Researchers' fieldwork accounts typically deal with such matters as how the hurdles blocking entry were successfully overcome and the emergent relationships cultivated and maintained during the course of the research: the emotional pains of this work are rarely mentioned.

Over the years, emotions have been explored in many different disciplines including anthropology, psychology and sociology. In sociology, emotions have been explored at length (see for example Bendelow & Williams, 1998; Denzin, 1984; Dunscombe & Marsden, 1996; Hochschild, 1983; James, 1989). Today we are witnessing a move away from viewing writing about emotions in research as a 'confessional tale' (Van Maanen, 1988:81) towards an acknowledgement and exploration of emotionality as a central tenet of the research process. This is particularly important when the research focuses on a sensitive topic that requires the researcher to investigate intimate aspects of people's lives.

In addition to researchers being more accepting of the emotional impact that their work can have on themselves, some argue that researchers should be taking their own emotions into account when designing and writing up research, as to ignore or downplay them may result in a distorted analysis (Kleinman & Copp, 1993; Ridge et al., 1999). However, it has been acknowledged that this is a very difficult thing to achieve. As William Shaffir and Robert Stebbins (1991:74) state, 'accounts of fieldwork are highly selective in what they reveal about the researcher's emotional experiences in the field'. Some researchers do acknowledge the importance of their own emotions but are often torn between presenting the emotions in the research and managing to present a certain level of objectivity to both their readers and their colleagues (Kleinman, 1991; Wilkins, 1993). Methodologically, feminist research has challenged the epistemological preferences of what has come to be called 'malestream' methodology by locating the researcher emotionally within the research.

Researchers have often reported feeling frustrated by the lack of discussion of the emotional nature of qualitative research. Ruth Wilkins, speaks of her frustration. She says, 'I consulted the approved academic and methodologic texts and was astonished at the intellectual cover-up of emotion . . . in the name of expert or academic knowledge' (Wilkins, 1993:94). Concern has been raised that if researchers openly express emotion their research may be seen as too emotional and subjective, thus devaluing the research (Kleinman, 1991). Kristen Swanson (1999), in her study of women who had experienced miscarriages, mentions the emotions of the participants at various stages in the research. However, she only refers to her own emotion at the very end of the paper stating that she 'couldn't help but emotionally respond' (Swanson, 1999:345). Comments like these are often relegated to the end of the paper where researchers briefly reflect on their own experiences. Researchers do not often report their own emotional states in much detail. This raises a number of questions for researchers who read these papers. They need to be able to ascertain what researchers mean when they say that they emotionally responded and how that response might have affected the research.

Over the past decade there has been growing awareness among some researchers that research *is* emotional and that researchers may not emerge largely unharmed and emotionally unaffected by their work. This awareness has culminated in a number of authors now explicitly referring to the emotional nature of their research (Bloor *et al.*, 2007; Campbell, 2002; Gilbert, 2001a; Goodrum & Keys, 2007; Harris & Huntington, 2001; Holland, 2007; Hubbard *et al.*, 2001; Johnson & Clarke, 2003; Lalor *et al.*, 2006; Lee-Treweek, 2000; Lee-Treweek & Linkogle, 2000b; McCosker *et al.*, 2001; Roberts, 2007; Spalek, 2007). Jennifer Harris and Annie Huntington (2001), in an edited book titled *The Emotional Nature of Qualitative Research*, highlight that all aspects of our lives have an emotional component. They include research or the 'academic production process' as one of those aspects and actively encourage researchers to take account of research as an emotional process. While many of these authors are including some emotional aspects of their work in their writing, a comprehensive examination of the emotional aspects of qualitative research, from the perspective of the researcher, has not been undertaken.

Qualitative research is an emotional activity and researchers need to be aware of the emotional nature of the research and anticipate the effects that it may have on them and their participants. Many of the researchers we interviewed spoke about managing both their own emotions and the emotions of their participants throughout the research process. This management can be examined using the theory of 'emotional labour' or 'emotion work' (Hochschild, 1983).

Emotion work theory

The terms 'emotional labour' and 'emotion work' are often used interchangeably in the literature. Initially, these two concepts were developed by Arlie Hochschild (1983:7) to mean different things as identified by the following definitions of the two terms. She says that 'emotional labour is sold for a wage', whereas 'emotion work' relates to the management of feelings done in private. Later, Nicky James (1989) used the term 'emotional labour' to describe any type of labour that involves dealing with other people's feelings. The core component of this type of labour is that you must be undertaking a regulation of your own feelings (James, 1989). Therefore, although Arlie Hochschild initially used the term 'emotional labour' to refer to emotional management during work done for a wage, it is now widely used to refer to any type of labour that involves the regulation of feelings.

The term 'emotion work' is generally used to refer to the work involved in 'dealing with other peoples emotions' (James, 1989:16). It has also been used to help define the work that people do on their own emotions in order to ensure that they are in line with the socially accepted 'feeling rules' – the rules that 'govern how people try to feel or not feel in ways which are appropriate to the situation' (Hochschild, 1979:552).

Arlie Hochschild (1983) estimated that approximately one-third of all jobs require substantial amounts of emotional labour and that women are more likely to hold such jobs than men. She stipulated that jobs requiring emotional labour involved face-to-face or voice-to-voice contact with members of the public. In a later examination of occupations requiring emotional labour (based on Hochschild's definition), Ronnie Steinberg and Deborah Figart (1999:16) found that jobs that require emotional labour have two defining characteristics. Firstly, 'they require contact with other people external to or within the organization, usually involving face-to-face or voice-to-voice interaction'. Secondly, emotional labour 'requires a worker to produce an emotional state in another person while at the same time managing one's own emotions'. This definition of emotional labour does not include the exchange of labour for a wage as one of its defining characteristics.

Since Hochschild's study of the emotional labour of flight attendants, many other authors have identified and examined the emotion work required of various other service professionals. Much of the early empirical research into emotional labour focused on various front-line service type occupations (see for example Ashforth & Humphrey, 1993; Van Maanen, 1990b; Van Maanen & Kunda, 1989) and workers' experiences of managing both their own emotions and the emotions of those they served. In addition to these studies others have been conducted with supermarket clerks (Tolich, 1993), clerical workers (Rogers, 1995; Wichroski, 1994), nurses and care assistants

(Aldridge, 1994; James, 1989, 1993; Lee-Treweek, 1996; Meerabeau & Page, 1998; O'Brien, 1994; Small, 1995; Smith, 1991, 1992), retail assistants (Godwyn, 2006), teachers (Nias, 1996), and the concept has been applied to the work of beauty therapists (Sharma & Black, 2001) and other professional groups (Harris, 2002; Pierce, 1999; Wharton, 1993). A number of researchers have attempted to quantify the number of occupations involving 'emotional labour'. Paula England (1992:62) identified 58 occupations that required 'an application of social skills to activities providing a service to customers or clients'.

Stephen Fineman (1993) has also examined emotional labour in organizations by bringing together a number of authors from disciplines such as sociology, psychology, criminology and organizational management. He feels that all organizations are 'emotional arenas' and further calls for the 'humanizing' and 'emotionalizing' of organizations (Fineman, 1993), thus opening the way for all workers to consider the 'emotional labour' required in undertaking their daily work.

It is clear from the research that has been done thus far, that emotional labour is a component of many different occupations, occurring in differing degrees. One occupation that has received limited attention is qualitative social research. The task of undertaking research has received only scant attention in the literature despite the suggestion by Susan Kleinman and Martha Copp that emotion work theory may also be applicable to researchers in the social sciences. Kleinman and Copp (1993:2) provide a detailed discussion of researchers' emotions highlighting that:

As members of the larger discipline, fieldworkers share a culture dominated by the ideology of professionalism or, more specifically, the ideology of science. According to that ideology, emotions are suspect. They contaminate research by impeding objectivity, hence they should be removed . . . fieldworkers, then, do emotion work (Hochschild, 1983) moulding their feelings to meet other's expectations.

Although research work does fit the criteria for emotion work that has been put forward by authors such as Hochschild (1983), James (1989), Kleinman and Copp (1993) and Steinberg and Figart (1999), undertaking research is still largely absent from classifications of occupations requiring emotion work. Very few authors have considered researchers when identifying those occupations that may be undertaking emotional labour. One exception is the work undertaken by Rebecca Campbell (2002) who applied the concept of research as emotional labour to her study with a small number of rape researchers. Campbell (2002) acknowledged that while researchers are not service professionals like those included in some of the early studies of emotion work (Hochschild, 1983), they do deal with people on a face-to-face basis and their involvement with research participants involves a considerable amount of personal interaction. While this was an important step in the process of understanding how research might affect researchers the concept has not been widely applied to researchers working in sensitive research areas.

In acknowledging the importance of emotions in the research process, we must also challenge the dominance of the Western philosophical tradition that judges emotions to be anathema to academic research. Arlie Hochschild (1983:22) focuses on the role of emotion for understanding the social world when she says that 'we infer other people's viewpoints from how they display feeling'. An emotional 'way of knowing' has often been contrasted with an objective, scientific approach. However, we think it is more appropriate for qualitative researchers to see their emotional and cognitive functions as inseparable from each other. Qualitative research on sensitive topics is a subjective experience that requires researchers to engage intellectually and emotionally with their participants, thus requiring simultaneous thinking and feeling.

In support of this, a number of authors argue strongly for emotions to be central to the research process (Ellis, 1991; Ellis & Bochner, 1999; Game, 1997; Hochschild, 1983). Ann Game (1997) also argues for sociologists to recognize and acknowledge the affective component of their work. She highlights that emotions enable us to make sense of and relate to our physical, natural and social worlds. Ruth Wilkins (1993:97) also speaks about what she terms 'the intellectual cover-up of emotion, intuition, and human relationships in the name of expert or academic knowledge'. However, we argue that it is appropriate for qualitative researchers to see their emotional and cognitive functions as inseparable from each other, and that emotions should be central to the research process (Ellis, 1991; Ellis & Bochner, 1999; Game, 1997; Hochschild, 1983; Roberts, 2007). It is clear that the theory of emotion is relevant to the work undertaken by qualitative researchers.

Showing emotion

A number of researchers have reported a range of differing emotions that they experienced while undertaking research on sensitive topics (Burr, 1995; Cannon, 1989; Cowles, 1988; Ellingson, 1998; Ellsberg *et al.*, 2001; Gilbert, 2001b; Goodrum & Keys, 2007; Higgins, 1998; Johnson & Clarke, 2003; Lalor *et al.*, 2006; Rowling, 1999). Some acknowledge openly crying with the participants in the interview (Burr, 1995; Liamputtong Rice, 2000; Matocha, 1992), while others talk of their emotions being pent up and released once they got home after the interview (Campbell, 2002; Gair, 2002). Some researchers have reported that undertaking sensitive research can be an emotionally distressing experience (Campbell, 2002; Cannon, 1992; Dunn, 1991; Gair, 2002; Rowling, 1999) often leaving them feeling quite drained.

Researchers also use emotional language when they speak of how they were affected in the field. For example, Dunn (1991:390) tells how she was 'choked with emotion' and Louise Rowling (1999:172) speaks of having 'tears in my eyes'. Researchers who are interacting with people undergoing particularly traumatic life experiences or who are in difficult situations do report feeling quite distressed by the situations of their participants (Warr, 2004).

While recounting their experiences of undertaking sensitive research many of the researchers that we interviewed spoke at length about their own emotions throughout the research experience. Although the emotions of study participants are often referred to in research literature (see for example Burr, 1995; Cameron, 1993; Cannon, 1989; Cowles, 1988; Demi & Warren, 1995; Draucker, 1999), it appears that researchers have been given little opportunity to talk about the emotions they experience as part of conducting research.

Many of the researchers we interviewed reported that they became emotionally overwhelmed during the research, stating that this was often directly attributable to the participants becoming emotional.

I cried pretty much the whole way through it because once she got upset it was impossible not to be upset you know.

. . . seven no it's eight – eight out of ten people I interview cry and they cry sometimes uncontrollably, it's a very sad thing to talk about . . . and how can you, as a person not get caught up in those feelings of sadness.

Researchers working in sensitive areas may encounter many different emotionally disturbing situations; for example, they may be confronted by a participant who is experiencing some type of psychological distress that may require some kind of support from the researcher, or they may be confronted with a participant who is emotionally distraught throughout the interview. Both of these situations require emotion work from the researcher.

Many of the researchers we interviewed spoke of emotion-generating situations. For example, a participant's story may evoke strong reactions from the researcher because it reminds the researcher of their own personal experiences or they may empathize with the participant's story. As outlined earlier, the ability to be empathetic is one of the main skills needed to undertake qualitative research (Liamputtong & Ezzy, 2005). While being empathetic it is often difficult not to get drawn into the emotion, especially when face to face with another person who is experiencing emotion. Some researchers do not attempt to hold back, or manage their emotions during the interview, instead preferring to become part of the experience themselves.

I just let em cry, cry with them, you know reach out and hold their hand, look at them, cry with them.

Although some researchers felt that open emotional displays like crying were problematic, others felt that becoming openly emotional was an important aspect of the research, signalling that the researcher had connected in a very personal and emotional way with the story that the participant was telling.

I become emotional, perhaps I cry but it's really not a bad thing – it tells me that I have connected. I have got to the essence of their story and they have told it so well that I can feel their pain.

Some of the researchers we interviewed were concerned about becoming emotional throughout the research as they felt that they were going against the 'rules' of how researchers were supposed to behave in a research encounter and whether becoming emotional while undertaking research was the 'right' thing to do. This was often strongly related to how they had been socialized as researchers.

Sometimes I think I would be better at this if I was a robot, a robot that had no capacity to feel anything – that would probably make my life much easier.

Some felt that, because it was not appropriate to be openly emotional during the interview, it was preferable to hold on until the interview was complete.

. . . and all I'm doing is trying really hard to try and hold back the tears myself.

I mean I burst into tears when I got out to the car – it was enormously distressing to watch this person in such distress when what you were seeing was enormous compassion struggling with deep ignorance and poor education and training and not knowing what to do with it.

This holding of emotion often left researchers feeling frustrated, which in turn often led to a release of emotion after the research.

I remember one night going to bed and I cried myself to sleep I was totally overwhelmed by the sadness of her story.

It's like you are allowed to 'feel' once the interview is over and you have the space to process your own feelings after the interview.

Emotions and academia

Part of this suppression of 'inappropriate' emotion may relate to notions about rigour in carrying out research. Sherryl Kleinman (1991) articulates a concern that if she were to really express her feelings and emotions she may be sending the wrong message (to her mainly quantitative colleagues), that field research was highly emotional and subjective and thus untrustworthy.

While authors like Liz Stanley and Sue Wise (1983) assert that research is more than an academic exercise, this is not often reflected in the literature. The foundation for academia is what could be termed 'proper science' and writing about one's own emotions throughout a research project is liable to be seen as not 'scientific' (Stanley & Wise, 1990). As students, researchers and professionals, we are products of a long process of socialization into academic life, often heavily reliant on the value of science and objectivity above all else. The difficulties associated with this have been acknowledged by Gill Hubbard, Kathryn Backett-Milburn and Debbie Kemmer (2001:135), who state that:

The challenge therefore is how we can construct meaning and develop understanding and knowledge in an academic environment that, on the whole, trains researchers to be objective and 'extract out' emotion?

The difficulties that researchers have in speaking about their own emotions in their research may be borne from this. Marcia Bellas (1999:104) argues that there are explicit occupational codes of conduct operating within academia that have led to the assumption that:

at first glance, research appears to involve little emotional labor relative to teaching and service. This perception stems from the strong association between science and objectivity, as well as the view that emotions are an impediment or contaminant to the scientific process.

Dealing with emotions generated in sensitive research can be difficult for researchers socialized in traditional methodologies that describe research in terms that relate to thinking, not feeling. Some feminist scholars have challenged this by arguing that feelings, like beliefs and values, shape the research and are a natural part of the process (Campbell & Wasco, 2000). The process of undertaking research on a sensitive topic must explicitly link emotion with knowledge, accepting that we cannot have one without the other (DeVault, 1997; Ellis, 1991; Fonow & Cook, 1991; Jaggar, 1989; Wilkins, 1993). Ann Game (1997) also argues that we must recognize that emotion plays a role in knowing the world and that knowledge then, is not something objective and removed from our bodies. She makes the point that emotions are the means by which we make sense of, and relate to, our physical, natural and social worlds. In this sense, emotion has particular epistemological significance as we can only truly 'know' through our experiencing something emotionally. Research, and particularly qualitative research, requires a combination of both technical skills and emotion work (Kleinman & Copp, 1993; Young & Lee, 1996; Campbell, 2002). It has been stated that this type of emotion work is often downgraded and seen as a poor substitute for the more technical skills (Kleinman & Copp, 1993), resulting in researchers not having the necessary skills to undertake emotion work.

Given this, it is not surprising that 'scientists (including social scientists) are trained to suppress emotions' (Bellas, 1999:104). Similarly, Pierre Bourdieu (1988) asserts that certain bodies of knowledge are reproduced through the training and professional socialization process (see also Calhoun, LiPuma & Postone, 1992). Bourdieu refers to the 'habitus' as having an influence on organizational culture. Habitus, argues Bourdieu, reflects the habitual patterns within an organization that seek to generate particular cultural patterns (Bourdieu & Wacquant, 1992). The process of academic socialization is often a very long one for researchers, with many of them having years of undergraduate and postgraduate work before coming to research positions. Throughout this early part of their research careers, academics develop certain patterns of behaviour. It could be argued that one of the key features of the academic habitus is the suppression of emotion. This has contributed to researchers being either unable or unwilling to talk about the emotional impact of the research that they conduct.

Other authors have also expressed their concern about the suppression of the emotional aspects of the knowledge production process (Game & Metcalfe, 1996). They remind us that much of the knowledge produced in the academic setting is strictly limited by publishers, researcher committees, funders and journal editors, and this process often results in the suppression or omission of the emotional aspects of the work in order to get it published (Game & Metcalfe, 1996).

Researchers' willingness to acknowledge the emotional nature of the work that they do may also reflect the gendered nature of emotion (Jaggar, 1989; Lupton, 1998). Allison Jaggar (1989:145) alerts us to the gendering of emotion:

Not only has reason been contrasted with emotion, but it has also been associated with the mental, the cultural, the universal, the public and the male, whereas, emotion has been associated with the irrational, the physical, the natural, the particular, the private and of course the female.

While the numbers of female researchers that we interviewed was higher (2:1) than the numbers of males, the gender balance generally reflected that of the disciplines involved. Female faculty members and women students tend to be concentrated in those fields where the expectations for emotional labour are the greatest (such as humanities, education, social work, nursing, public health), whereas the men are concentrated in those fields that could be defined as being unemotional (engineering, biological sciences, information technology) (Bellas, 1999).

One researcher we interviewed expressed his own theory about why the emotional aspects of research are not reported.

It is quite threatening for academics because academics are supposed to be professional and you are supposed to know everything . . . in qualitative research this is harder because here you're admitting that in fact you know less than you ever did and that your emotional reactions are pointing to issues and although your emotional reactions are pointing to important things in the data that you're linking into, they are also pointing to things that you haven't resolved in your own life and academics aren't very good at that, academics are very good at living in their heads.

In a sense this researcher felt that showing the emotional side of his work would in effect make him more vulnerable and open to judgements from his colleagues (mainly male quantitative researchers) about the scientific value of the knowledge that he was creating. He felt that the fact that he was undertaking mainly qualitative research compounded this.

The female researchers we interviewed were more inclined to report their own emotions than were their male counterparts. This disparity could be seen as a reflection of the gendering of emotional displays. Hochschild (1990) asserts that women are expected to undertake more emotion management than men, both at work and at home, rendering them more open to discussions of emotion. Previous research has shown that even within the same occupations, women are expected to perform more emotional labour than men (James, 1992; Wharton & Erickson, 1993; Wichroski, 1994). Given that qualitative research on sensitive topics is undertaken by both women and men it is important that both feel supported and able to talk about the emotional nature of undertaking research.

Emotions and embodied research

If we accept that qualitative research work can be emotion work we must also accept the embodied nature of the work. We cannot be emotionally involved in our research, showing emotion or feeling emotion, without using our bodies. Some researchers we interviewed reported showing an outward sign of emotion (crying) while others reported holding onto emotion until another point in time (see earlier discussion). Showing emotion at the point that it was felt and holding onto it until later both require some type of bodily action. Michelle Rosaldo (1984:143) illustrates this embodiment of emotion by stating that, 'emotions are thoughts somehow 'felt' in flushes, pulses, 'movements' of our lives. Minds, hearts, stomachs, skin. They are *embodied* thoughts'. By thinking of emotion in terms of an embodied experience we are able to see how our emotions are often displayed in an embodied way. Similarly, Carolyn Ellis and Arthur Bochner (1999) argue that researchers need to continually attend to their own emotions as a central part of research.

Maurice Merleau-Ponty (1962) was one of the first to write about embodied experiences, positing that through our bodies we come to know and understand other people. If we experience a strong physical sensation (such as crying) then the sensation (the bodily feeling) of that emotion captures our attention. He asserts that in order for something to be defined as an embodied experience it must also be a sensory experience that involves hearing, seeing and feeling, which helps us to know that something has taken place. Patricia Benner (2000:13) also focuses on the embodied nature of experience, stating that 'embodied understandings are really holistic impressions based on the ability of the individual to interpret contextual, historical and personal meanings associated with bodily responses'. Thus, in research, like in any other human interaction, our bodies know in an immediate way what has taken place (Williams & Bendelow, 1998). In order to participate in the world of other people we must use our own bodies, feeling with our bodies as we come to understand the experiences of others (Benner, 2000; Merleau-Ponty, 1962; Williams & Bendelow, 1998).

If we consider a research interview to be an embodied experience we can see how researchers use their bodies as part of that experience and how the feelings and emotions they experience help them to better understand the world of the participant. Many of the researchers we interviewed recounted their experiences of research using vivid imagery to describe both the person they were interviewing and their own feelings during that interview. In acknowledging that this research is often emotional we are also acknowledging that emotions are displayed bodily.

When she told me her story, so much detail, so sad, I felt my body tense up, feelings of anger, nausea . . . to think that someone could do that to another human being.

Listening to her talk, hearing her voice warble as she recounted her experience, I felt hot, somehow flustered, this was raw and I could tell.

I can still see her face to this day, she was so young, I could feel the paper in my hands shaking . . . a tremble in my voice as I tried not to show her how shocked I was.

I knew that my face was going red, flushed and hot . . . a lump in my throat making it hard to swallow, he had been so hurt, hurt by people that should have cared.

Drawing on Maurice Merleau-Ponty and his work in the study of emotions, Sue Cataldi (1993:63) suggests that emotion connects us to other people and puts us in touch. She refers to the tactile aspect of feeling an emotion:

There are tactile dimensions to emotional feelings and emotional dimensions to tactile ones. To say that we have been 'touched' . . . is synonymous with saying that we have been emotionally affected.

Similarly, many of the researchers we interviewed relayed feelings of being 'touched' by the stories of others, retelling how different people managed to 'touch' them in a very personal way.

That story, so beautifully told, touched me in many ways. It opened my eyes and my heart to the horror of some people's lives.

I was really touched by her story, she was so little and it must have been so hard, it made me think of my own children and what if it had been them?

In the above quotes the researchers talk about being 'touched', which includes some type of felt emotional response, either as the story was being told, or later on. These embodied responses serve to remind us to pay attention to how doing research might affect us emotionally. Embodied responses like those mentioned above are markers of meaning from which researchers can learn. By taking some time out to reflect on these physical and emotional aspects of research we might be better prepared both to undertake the research and to look after our own health while we are doing so.

Doing 'emotion work' in research

If we acknowledge that qualitative research is an embodied experience that requires some level of emotion work then we need to think about how we actually do emotion work and what that might mean. One aspect of emotion work is the management of emotion. Arlie Hochschild (1998:9) defines emotion management as 'an effort by any means, conscious or not, to change ones feeling or emotion'. As part of the emotion work that we do while undertaking qualitative research we manage our own feelings and outward displays of emotion. This is what Hochschild calls 'emotion management' and it is an integral part of the emotion work process.

Part of the embodied experience combined with the management of emotion often undertaken during this type of research can result in researchers giving an outward bodily display that is in conflict with their true feelings at the time.

I could feel myself physically reacting to her description, at times I felt physically ill while she recounted her story and I found myself, I mean I had to be very, very conscious of how I physically reacted, how I reacted to her at the time, my posture and so on, I had to be careful that I didn't make any judgments by looking horrified.

I nodded to let her know that I was listening but all the while I was feeling ill, in my head I was telling her to stop, wanting her to stop talking, but I kept on smiling and nodding.

This active management of feelings is central to research on sensitive topics as researchers often change the way they would normally act while engaged in research. One researcher shared her experience of managing her emotions.

Well I don't know how I did do it, because normally I am one of those people who cry fairly easily but I felt that it was important to maintain some sort of distance from them and I tried really hard, steeling myself a little bit and reminding myself that I didn't want that to happen [becoming emotional].

Many of those we interviewed spoke about the value of being professional, which involved not showing any outward signs of emotion. They referred to their ability to stay 'detached' from the research as offering them some protection from becoming emotional during the research. One researcher spoke of how she manages to be professional.

I do not react, don't show emotion, be professional – and remember that you are working and the people you are interviewing probably expect you to do that – they don't expect you to break down in the interview.

This quote is an example of a researcher managing their feelings and making sure that their bodily display does not match the felt emotion. It highlights the importance that some researchers place on being professional, which may include having to mask a felt emotion in order to manage how they display their emotion to the participant.

Sources of emotion work in research

Marcia Bellas (1999:104) states that, 'Despite the emphasis on emotional detachment and neutrality, researchers can become deeply involved in their subjects' lives, particularly when there is sustained contact between researchers and subjects'. Some of the difficulties of fieldwork have been attributed to the perils of undertaking a constant 'management of self'. According to William Shaffir, Robert Stebbins and Alan Turowetz (1980:iv):

> The intensity of the fieldwork process is typically accompanied by a psychological anxiety resulting in a continuous presentation and management of self when in the presence of those studied.

When recounting their experiences some of the researchers we interviewed talked about how they undertook a constant management of self in the research, especially in situations where there was a high level of expressed emotion: that is, people crying or feeling angry. As we outlined earlier, sensitive qualitative research is intimate and often goes into private spaces; often researchers are with people who may be experiencing difficulties in their lives (for example, victims of violence or those with cancer or drug dependency). By applying some of the definitions of emotion work and emotional labour provided by the different authors (Hochschild, 1983; James, 1989; Steinberg & Figart, 1999; Wharton, 1999) to the work of researchers, it is possible to build up a picture of what emotion work in research might consist of.

As discussed in Chapter 3, one of the most important preliminaries to undertaking qualitative research on a sensitive topic is the establishment of rapport. In order to establish rapport, researchers actively seek to make participants feel relaxed and comfortable enough to share their own experiences (Liamputtong, 2007). Establishing rapport often requires researchers to manage both their own emotions and those of the participants. This is a particularly important aspect of sensitive research due to the intimate nature of the research topics. As Hubbard, Backett-Milburn and Kemmer (2001:134) acknowledge, 'if it is important for the research project to encourage respondents to 'open up' about sensitive issues, then researchers need to find strategies to manage emotion'. Researchers need to find strategies to manage not only the emotions of the participants but also their own emotions. They will often get involved in sharing stories about themselves and listening to stories about participants as part of this process. Researcher self-disclosure (Liamputtong, 2007) was often reported by the researchers we interviewed with the hope of somehow creating a 'level playing field' for participants. This self-disclosure often required emotion work by the researchers, with many reporting feeling uncomfortable about having told participants personal things about themselves.

Other aspects of research that require emotion work include the management of the relationship with the participant, including leaving the relationship, and the management of self throughout the research. As we outlined in the previous chapter, the boundaries between researchers and participants often become blurred in this type of research and may require a considerable amount of emotion work from researchers to effectively manage them (Dickson-Swift *et al.*, 2006).

Consequences of doing emotion work

Arlie Hochschild (1983) refers to the 'human costs' of emotional labour, including burn-out to feeling phony, guilt and self-blame. Researchers may encounter emotionally disturbing situations throughout their data collection, such as witnessing someone who is in acute psychological distress or crying uncontrollably. Being confronted by these types of reactions from research participants may compel researchers to reflect on aspects of their own lives, which can in turn be an emotional experience. A number of the researchers we interviewed reflected on aspects of their own lives after being involved in qualitative research interviews. One researcher recounted how listening to a story about the impact of having a baby die reminded her about the death of her own baby.

I sort of had been pushing that away and not thinking about for the last ten years – thinking 'I'm over it – its gone' and when I'm hearing all this stuff I'm thinking 'Oh my god I felt that too', but I've been avoiding this for well sort of, sort of successfully for nearly ten years and now when I do this research it is all coming back – the research is bringing it back so that's when I decided to see the therapist and it's been good just to explore the issues that come out in my interviews and in myself too.

Much of the previous research on emotion work and emotional labour has focused on the potential negative consequences of that labour for the psychological health and well-being of the employees. For example, Hochschild (1983) reported that emotional labour could be linked to such problems as drug and alcohol abuse. In her research with flight attendants, she asserted that having to perform emotional labour had the potential to cause alienation and estrangement from genuine feelings and in doing so had detrimental consequences for psychological well-being. The pressures of research can have some 'detrimental effects on health and may lead to anxiety, alcohol abuse, depression and other problems' (Roberts 2007:46). Some of the consequences of emotion work for researchers were identified by those we interviewed. A number reported difficulties sleeping, anxiety, gastrointestinal upsets and depression similar to those previously reported in the literature.

Other authors have reported that the relationship between emotional labour and well-being is not as clear as that provided by Hochschild (1983).

Amy Wharton's (1993) study of emotional labour with employees in different job categories in a bank and a hospital showed no evidence that workers who perform emotional labour were more likely to suffer from emotional exhaustion. Instead Wharton (1993) found that emotional labour could be positively related to job satisfaction. This is in direct contrast to the findings of Hochschild (1983). However, Blake Ashforth and Ronald Humphrey (1993) suggest that emotional labour may actually help people to psychologically distance themselves from unpleasant situations. The researchers that we interviewed used a number of strategies to distance themselves from the data, including reminding themselves that the research was not about them and that they are professional researchers and, therefore, should not get involved.

Researchers working on sensitive topics are at risk of becoming overwhelmed and physically and mentally exhausted when undertaking research interviews. This sense of exhaustion may relate to the fact that many feel quite overwhelmed by the nature of the data.

. . . by the time I got home I was just like exhausted, just emotionally exhausted.

I was just interviewing all day, I would have done more than five interviews – I was just interviewing all day, by myself and I was really buggered[1], yeah I was had it.

I found it really emotionally draining . . . it got to the point where I had to allocate time . . . I can go and do the interview in the morning but then I will have to block out the rest of the day because after that I need to go home and I need to digest what has happened . . . go through it in my head.

Emotional exhaustion has been reported by a range of researchers working on sensitive topics (see for example Alexander *et al.*, 1989; Goodrum & Keys, 2007; Gregory *et al.*, 1997; Letherby, 2000; McCosker *et al.*, 2001). Goodrum and Keys (2007:256) explain how they felt 'burdened by the weight of participants' sadness' and that this led them to consider their own well-being. This emotional exhaustion often leaves researchers feeling physically tired, especially if they have been involved in a particularly emotional interview.

. . . and the ones where there was this overwhelming sense of hopelessness, the ones that left you feeling like you have just run the marathon – you know and after one of those, shaping up for the next one was a bit like '. . . agh . . . I hope this one's not too sad'.

Emotional exhaustion is a specific stress-related reaction and has been identified as one of the key components of burn-out (Maslach, 1982). Emotional exhaustion is characterized by feeling emotionally overextended and depleted (Maslach, 1998). Christina Maslach's (1982) research suggests that frequent face-to-face encounters with people (especially interactions that are

---

[1] The term 'buggered' is an Australian colloquialism for exhausted.

particularly emotionally intense) are associated with high levels of emotional exhaustion. This is important since researchers doing repeated face-to-face interviews with little time in between to debrief and recover may be at risk of emotional exhaustion.

Emotional and physical exhaustion of researchers has been previously reported in the literature (Cannon, 1992; Johnson & Clarke, 2003; McCosker *et al.*, 2001; Parker & Ulrich, 1990); however, much of this evidence is anecdotal. The emotional and physical exhaustion that accompanies the research experience is not always related to the data that is being collected, but it may be related to the researcher's reaction to the data. For some researchers, undertaking research in a specific area forced them to confront similar experiences in their own lives. As one researcher says:

I have found this research really hard, both mentally and emotionally. It has made me confront a lot of things in my own life and I haven't dealt with them yet.

Many of the researchers we interviewed reflected on their choice of research topic stating that in many cases their topic selection came directly from their own life experiences.

I mean one interesting thing about academia is that people tend to research things where they have got unresolved issues . . . we all do that!

It may be important for researchers to consider how they became interested in certain topics. John and Lyn Lofland (1995:13) state, 'it is often said among sociologists that, as sociologists, we 'make problematic' in our research matters that are problematic in our lives'. If we undertake research on topics that resonate with issues in our own lives, it is possible that undertaking the research will have some type of emotional impact on us.

. . . its not just about saturation of when you don't get new themes . . . it's about your saturation as well – how much you can actually take and I could not, could not have fronted for another one of those interviews.

That 30 year old that I was telling you about who was so abused by his parents – he stands out as one of those guys that I haven't been really able to exorcise from my mind you know. Every now and again I cast him a thought because I see him on the streets occasionally because it brings it all back to me.

Researchers working with particularly traumatic material may be subject to a degree of vicarious traumatization (McCann & Pearlman, 1990; Schauben & Frazier, 1995). Vicarious traumatization has been defined as the process by which individuals listening to and working with the traumatic experiences of others begin to experience the effects of trauma themselves. Although this concept has been applied mainly to counsellors and therapists, it has been argued that the concept is an 'equally valid phenomenon for all human service workers who are exposed in a secondary fashion to client trauma'

(Lonne, 2003:285). Researchers working on sensitive topics, although not human service workers, are often exposed in a secondary fashion to the trauma experienced by others.

A few of the researchers we interviewed admitted to becoming quite withdrawn from family, friends and colleagues while they were involved in the interview stage of their research.

I didn't want to talk to anyone, see anyone; I had so much going on in my head, trying to make sense of all that hurt . . . I guess it took me a few months to deal with all that.

. . . and I slept of the edge of the bed, I didn't sleep right next to him for a period of time. I don't remember how long . . . it was really weird, cause I just didn't want to be near him in a sense.

Researchers involved in research on sensitive topics may experience feelings of exhaustion, guilt, anxiety, disconnection from family and friends, and social withdrawal. These are all symptoms of vicarious traumatization (Dane, 2000; Sexton, 1999). While it is clear that not all researchers experience research in the same way, the fact that participating in research can have a number of physical and psychological effects on researchers needs to be acknowledged.

The value of taking emotions (both of researchers and of respondents) into account when designing, carrying out and writing up research has been recognized by Jennifer Harris and Annie Huntington (2001:131) who state that:

if we take emotions and emotional labour seriously into account, then we open a space within which we can explore practical strategies to work with our emotional responses. In addition, we bring to light aspects of our experience that may be particularly problematic for novice researchers or those engaged with substantive topics that are likely to engender strong reactions (for example, sexual abuse of children).

If we are going to advocate for the acknowledgement of researchers undertaking emotion work in research then we must also consider the types of support that may need to be made available to researchers. Many researchers we interviewed reported using informal support networks of colleagues, trusted friends and family members for support and debriefing throughout the research. This informal peer support is very important for researchers, particularly as the concept of emotion work is undervalued within the university culture. It has been previously reported that much of the discussion about emotions in research and how the researcher actually 'feels' in the process is often done informally at the photocopier, coffee machine or in the corridors (see Chapter 3) (Hubbard *et al.*, 2001). If we are to create a space for researchers to explore the emotional nature of the work that they do then we need to ensure that appropriate support is offered, both institutionally and individually, for researchers to do that.

Summary

It is clear from the discussion in this chapter that researchers undertake a significant amount of emotion work in their daily research activities. Qualitative researchers working on sensitive topics are advised to consider the emotion work involved in such research and as outlined here, and consider putting strategies for self-care, such as debriefing and peer mentoring and support, in place before beginning the research. Such self-protection strategies are outlined in more detail in Chapter 7.

Tutorial activities

(a) In this chapter we discussed how qualitative research on sensitive topics can be considered emotion work. What are the important criteria that define some occupations as emotion work? Consider your own area of research; what is the likelihood of participants becoming emotionally distressed during a research interview on this topic? How do you plan to deal with emotional responses from participants?

(b) What are the common signs of burn-out that you should be aware of in yourself and your colleagues?

SUGGESTED READING

Campbell, R. (2002). *Emotionally Involved: The Impact of Researching Rape.* New York: Routledge.

Carter, K. & Delamont, S. (eds.) (1996). *Qualitative Research: The Emotional Dimension.* Aldershot: Avebury.

Gilbert, K.R. (ed.) (2001). *The Emotional Nature of Qualitative Research.* London: CRC.

Goodrum, S. & Keys, J.L. (2007). Reflections on two studies of emotionally sensitive topics: bereavement from murder and abortion. *International Journal of Social Research Methodology,* **10**(4), 249–258.

Holland, J. (2007). Emotions and research. *International Journal of Social Research Methodology,* **10**(3), 195–209.

Hubbard, G., Backett-Milburn, K. & Kemmer, D. (2001). Working with emotions: issues for the researcher in fieldwork and teamwork. *International Journal of Social Research Methodology,* **4**(2), 119–137.

Lee-Treweek, G. & Linkogle, S. (eds.) (2000). *Danger in the Field: Risk and Ethics in Social Research.* London: Routledge.

Ramsay, K. (1996). Emotional labour and qualitative research: how I learned not to laugh or cry in the field. In E.S. Lyon & J. Busfield (eds.), *Methodological Imaginations.* Basingstoke: Macmillan.

Managing risks and ethics in research

6

Traditionally risk in universities has been seen in terms of threats from physical work and from accidents on campus; academic and research staff have not been 'risk assessed' in relation to social research activity. Notions about academic work as a pen-pushing middle class pursuit contribute to the under-recognition of the risks of social research.

(Lee-Treweek & Linkogle, 2000b:201)

While ethics committees and research supervisors are well versed in assessing risks to potential participants in sensitive research, the risks for the researchers and other members of the research team are often not considered. In this chapter we provide an overview of risk theory and examine risks in sensitive research. We offer some discussion regarding roles and responsibilities of risk assessment and management, and discuss ethical issues including confidentiality, anonymity and review the role of ethics committees in assessing potential harm to researchers. Based on evidence gained from researchers in the field, in this chapter we argue that there is currently insufficient recognition of the need for protection of researchers and other members of the research team involved in qualitative research on sensitive topics.

Theorizing risk

Monitoring of risk is a key aspect of modern society (Beck, 1992, 1994; Giddens, 1991, 1992, 1993), which has come to be known as a 'risk society' (Beck, 1992:5). Ulrich Beck (1992:5) states that risks 'only exist in terms of the (scientific or anti-scientific) knowledge about them. They can be changed, magnified, dramatized or minimized with knowledge, and to that extent they are particularly open to social definition and construction'. The concept of risk has become central to the way the social world is organized. Living and working in a 'risk society' encourages us to be more self-reflexive, examining the risks and hazards that impact on our everyday lives (Fox, 1998, 1999).

If we examine our current practices we may be able to raise awareness and encourage reflexivity, accountability and responsibility (Lupton, 2002). Since it appears possible to minimize risks with knowledge (Beck, 1992) it is important that we build knowledge about risk in research so that we can put in place strategies to deal with the risks that may arise. Nick Fox (1998; 1999) argues that risk is 'in the eye of the beholder' and that people who have not had the experience themselves may not see the risks. However, the people actually involved in the 'doing' see the risks as real. This is an interesting statement, for some academic researchers may think that arguing that research is risky is just being overly paternalistic or simplistic – but if risk is in the eye of the beholder then if that particular person sees it as a risky activity then that is all that is important (Fox, 1999). In the past few years there has been some debate about whose role it is to assess risk for researchers. Institutional ethics committees (IECs), supervisors, granting bodies, research-ers and the wider university sector all have a role to play (Bloor *et al.*, 2007; Dickson-Swift *et al.*, 2005; Dickson-Swift *et al.*, 2008; Lee-Treweek & Linkogle, 2000a).

Ethics in sensitive research

Conducting research on sensitive topics raises a number of specific ethical issues that require careful consideration (Lee-Treweek & Linkogle, 2000a; Lee, 1993). Researchers proposing a project that focuses on a sensitive topic need to be vigilant about confidentiality, privacy and anonymity. Geraldine Lee Treweek and Stephanie Linkogle (2000b:15) argue that researchers need to protect their research participants and that consideration of the ethics of gaining access to a person's private world and discussing painful experiences is necessary. Although ethical issues are important in all research, researchers involved in research on sensitive topics must be particularly cautious about confidentiality, informed consent and anonymity of their participants (Dickson-Swift, 2005).

Confidentiality and anonymity

The aim of confidentiality is to conceal the true identity of the participants (Christian, 2005) and most ethical codes require that researchers maintain confidentiality of participants (Liamputtong Rice & Ezzy, 1999; NHMRC, 1999, 2007). Maintaining confidentiality when carrying out qualitative research may be difficult because a great deal of qualitative data is collected during an interaction between researcher and participant (NHMRC, 1995, 2007). Researchers utilizing qualitative methods may use a number of strat-egies to ensure the anonymity of research participants, such as combining various parts of different participants' responses to research questions to build up a composite picture (Lincoln & Guba, 1985) or giving research sites a fictitious name (Melrose, 2002).

Many of the topics studied by qualitative researchers involve very small or very specific samples, such as members of one small ethnic group (Liamputtong Rice, 2000; Lipson, 1997) or particular geographical locations, which may complicate the process of maintaining anonymity (Hopkins, 1993; Nespor, 2000). Researchers need to take care that those people, or their town, or their group, cannot be identified by the research, while at the same time balancing the need to offer 'thick description' (Geertz, 1973:5) and accuracy. Some people may choose to participate in research on sensitive topics because of the promise of confidentiality and it has been highlighted that researchers must be 'up front' with potential participants if they cannot promise confidentiality (for example due to mandatory reporting laws) (Booth, 1999; Melrose, 2002). In her research with juvenile prostitutes in England and Wales, Margaret Melrose (2002:342) argues that due to the very sensitive nature of her research, it was important for her and the research team to promise confidentiality to the participants. The research team also anticipated that there might be some circumstances where confidentiality could not be guaranteed, particularly when there was an urgent threat to the safety or life of the participants. The potential participants were informed at the outset of the research about the conditions under which confidentiality may be breached.

Informed consent

Informed consent has been defined as:

the provision of information to participants, about the purpose of the research, its procedures, potential risks, benefits and alternatives so that the individual understands this information and can make a voluntary decision whether to enrol and continue to participate. (Emanuel, Wendler & Grady, 2000:2703)

Informed consent is a prerequisite for all research; however, gaining this consent in sensitive research is often fraught with difficulty (Lee, 1993; Liamputtong, 2007; Liamputtong & Ezzy, 2005; Renzetti & Lee, 1993). In order to assist researchers to ensure that there is true informed consent they are encouraged to assess their research against the criteria outlined by Charles Bosk (2002:S-65) summarized in Box 6.1.

Researchers seeking to gain informed consent from participants need to ensure that the potential participants fully understand what it means for them to participate in the study and that they have really consented to do so (Lipson, 1994). It is paramount that this informed consent is voluntary. Voluntary consent has been defined by Sieber (1992:26) as 'an on-going

> **Box 6.1** Four criteria for assessing informed consent in sensitive research
>
> - Disclosure – a full disclosure of the nature of research that will take place, including a warning of any potentially sensitive or emotional topics that will be covered.
> - Understanding – researchers must ensure that the potential participants fully understand what they are consenting to. This includes a complete outline of the roles and responsibilities of both researchers and participants including the demands, risks, inconveniences, discomforts and benefits that might be involved.
> - Voluntariness – participation needs to be voluntary and potential participants must have a specific agreement about what participation entails.
> - Competence – judging competence for consent is not always easy but researchers may need to discuss issues of competence with a third party (gatekeeper, family member etc.).

two-way communication process between subjects and the investigator, as well as specific agreement about the conditions of the research participation'. It is important for researchers to remember that there are often language and/or cultural barriers influencing an understanding of what participation in a research study may mean (Liamputtong, 2007).

Usually the informed consent agreement takes the form of a signed consent form; however, signed informed consent may not always be appropriate or achievable (Liamputtong, 2007; Liamputtong Rice, 1996; Lipson, 1994; Minichiello *et al.*, 2000). For example, 'when signed consent would jeopardise the well-being of the subject, when the research focuses on illegal or highly stigmatised aspects of the persons being studied' (Sieber, 1992:38) a signed informed consent may not be appropriate. Researchers working with migrant groups also report that written consent may be potentially intimidating and offensive (Hennings, Williams & Haque, 1996; Liamputtong Rice, 1996; Lipson & Meleis, 1989; Lipson, 1994). As pointed out by Jean Hennings and colleagues (1996:15) it is important for researchers working on sensitive research with immigrants to realize that 'in a culture where the spoken word is taken as a binding legal contract, to ask for signed consent would be to imply mistrust'. In some cases requesting signed informed consent may result in potential participants refusing to participate in the research. It may infringe on the well-being of some people who may fear reprisal for signing the form. Some groups of people will not give signed consent as they may be illiterate or unwilling to sign any official documents (Liamputtong, 2007; Liamputtong Rice, 1996). In some types of sensitive research it may be appropriate, and in some cases preferable, to obtain verbal consent and ensure a witness is available (Liamputtong Rice, 1996; Ringheim, 1995).

In order to obtain full informed consent researchers need to ensure that they provide a full disclosure of the nature of the research that will take place, including a warning about any potentially sensitive or emotional topics that will be covered. Potential participants also need to be aware that they are taking part in the study of their own free will and that they are free to withdraw from the study if they choose. Ringheim (1995:1694) argues that the notion of 'free will' is a cultural construct, which implies a level of personal autonomy and individual rights that can vary greatly across different societies. Researchers should ensure that all participants know that participation in the study is voluntary. This raises a number of important issues when using community gatekeepers to assist in gaining access to samples for sensitive research. Some participants may feel unable to refuse to participate if an important community leader or gatekeeper has given permission for the study to go ahead.

Risks and problems in sensitive research

Many of the risks inherent in sensitive research have been raised by a range of different authors (Campbell, 2002; Cannon, 1992; Dunn, 1991; Erlandson, Harris, Skipper & Allen, 1993; Etherington, 2007; Johnson & Clarke, 2003; Lipson, 1994; Renzetti & Lee, 1993; Smith, 1992). However, few have offered suggestions for researchers to assess and evaluate the problems that may arise. Joan Sieber (1993:19) argues that, 'the potential risks, sensitivities and benefits in sensitive research are the same as those in any social research, but greater in magnitude'. Prior to beginning recruitment and data collection most researchers have already submitted a proposal to a funding body or to an institutional ethics committee (IEC) explaining in detail how they will manage any possible risks to those they are hoping to study. However, 'the issue of their own or their co-researchers' safety and welfare needs are often thought through in a cursory manner or in an *ad hoc* contingent fashion once in the field' (Lee-Treweek & Linkogle, 2000b:1).

Many of the researchers that we interviewed felt that researchers should be encouraged to give more consideration to the risks inherent in research. Some spoke openly about the risks they faced in undertaking their research project, framing them in terms of both physical and emotional risks.

I think there is always a risk in this research. You have got to remember that sometimes we go into spaces in people's lives that others have not been and that has the potential to be risky, both physically if the environment is not a safe one, or emotionally if the research affects you in some way.

Physical risks

It is interesting to note that despite the length of time that researchers have been carrying out ethnographic/anthropological studies in settings that may be considered dangerous, on topics that may be considered sensitive, it is surprising that the literature outlining the possible physical risks researchers may face is so limited (Ferrell & Hamm, 1998; Lee-Treweek & Linkogle, 2000a; Lee, 1995).

In *Dangerous Fieldwork*, Raymond Lee draws a distinction between what he terms 'ambient' and 'situational danger' (Lee, 1995:3). He states that ambient danger is present in the actual setting and he uses the example of the dangers encountered by Brewer when he was studying policing in Northern Ireland (Lee, 1995:3). Ambient danger has also been identified in other studies, for example Ben Fincham's study of bicycle messengers in the United Kingdom (Fincham, 2006). Bicycle messengers are constantly faced with dangers in the setting of their day-to-day work. Situational danger, on the other hand, relates to danger arising out of the presence of a researcher that may provoke hostility, aggression or violence from those within the setting (see for example Lee-Treweek & Linkogle, 2000b; Lee, 1995; Schramm, 2005).

Many researchers have found themselves in situations where their physical safety is compromised (Campbell, 2002; Sampson & Thomas, 2003). Thankfully, reports of deaths to fieldworkers are relatively rare; however, there are many accounts of researchers spending time in settings that are particularly risky (for example undertaking research with drug users, streetworkers, criminals etc.). Gender may also have a role to play when assessing risk in research. The gender of a researcher may alter the situation in the field when considering well-being, and there have been reports of female researchers being exposed to sexual harassment and/or assault (Coffey, 1999; Moreno, 1995; Sampson & Thomas, 2003).

Emotional risks

As we discussed in Chapter 5, there is a possibility that researchers undertaking sensitive research may be exposed to emotional risk (Bloor *et al.*, 2007; Campbell, 2002; Dickson-Swift *et al.*, in press; Dunn, 1991; Gilbert, 2001b; Lee-Treweek, 2000; Malacrida, 2007; Milling-Kinard, 1996; Rosenblatt, 2001). Research work is often emotionally draining for researchers and if we are to think about the possibilities of researchers being in risky situations then we need to consider both physical and emotional risk. Research projects on sensitive topics involving interviews with victims of sexual abuse, cancer patients and bereaved children have all been examined in light of the emotional impact that the research had on the researcher (Burr, 1995; Campbell, 2002; Cannon, 1989; Grinyer, 2004; Rager, 2005a; Rowling, 1999; Scott, 1998; Wray *et al.*, 2007). The face-to-face nature of the qualitative research encounter, coupled with listening to the stories of others retold about grief, loss and sadness can clearly have some emotional costs for researchers.

The importance of assessing risk

Risk assessments in research have traditionally been limited to an examination of the risks to research *participants*. There is now growing acknowledgement that research can also pose risks to researchers (Bloor *et al.*, 2007; Dickson-Swift *et al.*, 2008; Lee-Treweek, 2000; Lee-Treweek & Linkogle, 2000a; Liamputtong, 2007; Social Research Association, 2006). In their edited book, *Danger in the Field: Risk and Ethics in Social Research*, Geraldine Lee-Treweek and Stephanie Linkogle (2000a) identify the need for academic researchers to consider the risks to themselves while undertaking fieldwork. They highlight that 'there are also issues arising out of risk management for academics and researchers, for instance we often study the risks to society, from ill health or crime, etc., yet we rarely consider the dangers involved in carrying out research' (Lee-Treweek & Linkogle, 2000a:9).

Historically, the focus of the IECs has been on protection of the participant, which is unarguably one of their main roles (Central Office for Research Ethics Commiittees (COREC), 2006; Dickson-Swift *et al.*, 2005; Mauthner *et al.*, 2002; Medical Research Council of Canada (MRC), National Science and Engineering Research Council of Canada (NSERC) & Social Science and Humanities Research Council of Canada (SSHRC), 1998; NHMRC, 1999, 2007; Sieber, 1993). However, the protection of the researcher is often left unassessed. While the IECs often require a detailed protocol outlining how the researchers will respond to potential psychological distress resulting from participation in an interview, IECs often fail to acknowledge that there is potential for psychological and/or physical harm to the others involved in the research process (Bloor *et al.*, 2007; Dickson-Swift *et al.*, 2005; McCosker *et al.*, 2001).

One of the researchers we interviewed raised the point that universities have an obligation to protect researchers from harm under 'duty of care' and occupational health and safety guidelines.

I think it's really important for them [universities] to remember that there is harm in research and if universities have a duty of care to their staff then it's part of occupational health and safety, it's part of mental health promotion.

Many of the researchers we interviewed spoke about the lengths that they went to, to satisfy the ethics committee about the safety of the participants; however, they also raised the point that they often did not think about the risks that they might face while they were involved in the research.

. . . you were that busy trying to assure everybody [on the ethics committee] that you weren't going to do any harm or whatever to the participants that you never got to think about yourself.

A narrow definition of risk to researchers is often provided in the ethics guidelines for undertaking human research (Dickson-Swift *et al.*, 2005).

This narrow definition tends to encourage researchers not to focus on risk to themselves, but only on those risks to the research participants (Bloor *et al.*, 2007; Dickson-Swift *et al.*, 2005). Researchers should be 'risk assessing' their research to ensure that the ethical mandate of 'do not harm' is being adhered to. Researchers should be considering this mandate for themselves as well as for their research participants. Milling-Kinard (1996:65) echoes the thoughts of many other authors when examining the role of the IEC in approving research:

> In order to gain approval for the use of human subjects in research, investigators must provide detailed methods for protecting subjects from harm. However, they are not required to consider the potentially negative effects of conducting research on the researchers themselves.

The National Health and Medical Research Council (NHMRC) in Australia, which is responsible for ethical conduct of all research involving humans, also alerts ethics committee members and researchers to consider some of the risks to researchers when it alerts researchers that:

> Interviews can also trigger feelings for the researcher. It is not uncommon for interviews to become confessionals for the participant . . . Adequate support for both researchers and participants should be available as needed. This might include debriefing for the interviewer and counselling for the participant, particularly in studies investigating sensitive areas such as physical or psychological trauma or abuse, death, dying and grief. These support strategies should also be available to both parties at the point of disengagement and termination of the research relationship. (NHMRC, 2002:E131)

So, while there is some recognition that participation in research may raise some difficulties for qualitative researchers, ethics committees have largely not adopted these assessments as part of their main role (Bloor *et al.*, 2007; Dickson-Swift *et al.*, 2005).

Concerns have been raised about the implications for ethics committees when assessing the risks to researchers (Kitson *et al.*, 1996; Langford, 2000). Issues mentioned include: personal safety of researchers, researchers coping with both their own and their participants' emotions, such as crying and anger throughout the interviews, and handling the problems that arise in the interviews. Gay Kitson and her colleagues (1996) felt that it was important to be 'up front' with the anticipated risks to the researcher and researched with the IEC and called for safeguards to be in place for 'all participants' (including researchers) in research. In order for researchers to be up front with the IEC about the risks to the researchers there is a need for committees to provide some type of guidelines for researchers to ensure that they have undertaken a thorough assessment of the potential risks of the research. While some may argue that extending the role of the IEC to also make assessments about harm to researchers may be unnecessarily paternalistic (Lee-Treweek &

Linkogle, 2000b; Orb, Eisenhauer & Wynaden, 2001), others would argue that research institutions have a 'duty of care' to all workers, including researchers (Dickson-Swift *et al.*, 2005).

It has previously been reported that researchers and transcribers undertaking research on sensitive issues such as domestic violence, for example, may experience physical and emotional symptoms including headaches, sleep disturbances and gastrointestinal upsets (Burr, 1995; Cowles, 1988; Etherington, 2007; Gregory *et al.*, 1997). Natalie Wray and colleagues (2007: 1397) spoke about their emotional overload and how it led them to experience 'frequent headaches, anxiety and panic, a 'foggy head', dizziness and nausea'. Heather McCosker and colleagues (2001) in their examination of the issues for researchers undertaking sensitive research, include issues for *all* those participating in the research including the researcher, research assistants, transcribers and other members of the research team. Pranee Liamputtong (2007) and Gay Kitson and colleagues (1996) have also discussed the importance of including both transcribers and researchers in the ethical assessment process.

Preparation for research

The exploratory nature of qualitative research means that researchers often go into a qualitative interview with very little control over the topics that will be discussed. Some researchers have raised the issue of feeling unprepared for undertaking research on a sensitive topic (Batchelor & Briggs, 1994; Johnson & Clarke, 2003; Kiesinger, 1998). Louise Rowling (1999:175) spoke of her frustration when she was researching loss and grief. She says:

Nothing that I read in planning this study prepared me for the emotionality of the research process. I read recommendations about how I should address confidentiality, harm, deception and privacy, but there was not much written on such things as the impact on the researcher of listening to people talk about their grief, their fears and anxieties, sometimes being expressed for the first time and in times of crisis.

Gayle Burr (1995:174) also felt very unprepared for undertaking a study with families of critically ill patients: 'my level of preparedness and skill was barely adequate for the depth of disclosure that sometimes occurred', she remarked. The sense of unpreparedness was particularly overwhelming for Christine Kiesinger (1998:73) who says that, 'none of my training, scholarship, or courses in the areas of ethnography, interactive interviewing, or qualitative research methods prepared me for the depth of emotionality . . .'. This point is echoed by Hubbard, Backett-Milburn and Kemmer (2001) who speak of their feelings of unpreparedness while undertaking an interview in which the respondent spoke of his father's death. They report the difficulties of seeing someone else crying and how that affected them in the interview.

Barbara Johnson and Jill Macleod Clarke (2003:423–424) report that the researchers they interviewed felt very unprepared for the situations in which they found themselves. They felt that in their preparation for research there had been a great deal of emphasis placed on things like accessing participants and gaining entry but 'little or no orientation to the kinds of difficulties and concerns that they might encounter during the research process'.

In sensitive research, the nature of the subject matter studied may have an isolating effect on the researcher (Campbell, 2002; Moran-Ellis, 1996). Studying emotionally demanding topics in unfamiliar environments without adequate space for reflection or opportunities to talk through the difficult issues faced by researchers can have a negative effect on researchers.

Researchers provide a space for participants to tell their story, and in that telling the researchers may be taken to places that they were not prepared for. Many of the difficulties reported by the researchers that we interviewed related to the emergent nature of qualitative research, which raises a number of issues regarding preparation for research.

Research is always unpredictable and often what you think might happen doesn't and something you hadn't prepared for will and because of that I think it probably is important for ethics committees to think about those sorts of things.

I think you never really know how it's going to go, you never really know what the people are going to be like or where it's going to head. It's qualitative and sometimes it can go to places where you didn't think you would go and they can sometimes be very intimate and dangerous, both for you the researcher and for the participants, you can't really think through all the possibilities.

You can never really know exactly the types of things that you as a researcher will be faced with in this type of research . . . things that really make you think, make you worry, make you sad . . . you can't prepare for all those.

The differences between the level of training, supervision and risk assessment undertaken by different types of researchers was evident.

You know if you were a scientist in a lab you would have heaps of training and supervision to make sure that you are mixing the chemicals properly, you wear safety glasses, coats and boots, but if you are a scientist in the field you pretty much make it up as you go along.

Many authors have commented that undertaking sensitive research requires more than just standard research training (Bloor *et al.*, 2007; Carter & Delamont, 1996; Driscoll, Hull, Mandryk *et al.*, 1997; Lee-Treweek & Linkogle, 2000b; Owens, 1996; Social Research Association, 2006). David Owens (1996:65) suggests that:

. . . an understanding of, and training in, basic counselling skills would be of help, not so that interviewers could become some kind of counsellor, but rather because many of those skills make one better equipped to deal with emotional interviews and remain professional in the face of displays of emotion and emotional requests for help.

Owens (1996:65) goes on to add that 'at the very least, knowledge of these skills can help ensure that well-intentioned but essentially amateur and ill-considered 'counselling' does not take place'. As discussed in Chapter 4, some of the researchers we interviewed felt that counselling skills were essential for this type of research, while others felt that possession of these skills only complicated the boundary issues inherent in sensitive research.

Universities (and research centres) have a duty of care to researchers (and participants) to ensure that they are not harmed in any way (physically or emotionally) from their participation in research. John Roberts and Teela Saunders (2005) have raised this issue observing that much qualitative research takes place in an academic environment where there should be a very clear structural context. Researchers are bounded by these institutions and must operate within their guidelines; reciprocally institutions have responsibilities towards 'their' researchers.

When the researchers we interviewed spoke about the possibility of risk to themselves they were asked whose responsibility it was to ensure the risks were minimized. While many of them stated that risk assessment and management were a joint responsibility of both the researcher and the super-visor, others felt that it was the role of the IEC. Given that not all researchers in this study had formal supervision arrangements in place (for example, senior researchers working in research institutions attached to universities) this is not surprising. The role of the IEC in assessing risk to researchers has been debated in the literature (Bloor *et al.*, 2007; Dickson-Swift *et al.*, 2005) and a number of the researchers we interviewed felt that there was a clear role for the IEC, with failure to recognize risk to researchers as a legitimate concern resulting in harm to researchers.

You know the ethics committee at the moment considers only the risks to the participants whereas I think there is risk for other people. I think there is risk for your supervisors, there is risk for the transcribers, anybody who actually has involvement with the research in any real sense – see my supervisors all said that they found reading my thesis for the first time really distressing because they couldn't believe that human beings could behave like the women reported they did.

I think it is an ethical issue that the ethics committee may allow research to go ahead that might damage the researcher. There is quite a lot of responsibility that should be put back onto the ethics committees and at present it is not there at all. We need to start questioning ethics committees because I think it is about the research and the whole process of the research, not just about one person, it's not just about the participants, it's often about us too.

While it is possible to argue that the responsibility for protecting researchers from harm while they are undertaking sensitive research lies with the super-visors or chief investigators, both the university and IEC also have a role to play.

One of the main issues is that, in research, people assume that if you hold an Honours, Masters or Doctoral degree that you have a certain level of competence in research. While this may be true when referring to the technical aspects of research, there are many other issues that need to be considered when the research topic is a sensitive one. How can we be sure that those whom we send out to do interviews on sensitive topics have any minimum level of competence in dealing with research participants who may be undergoing significant emotional reactions during the research? We cannot. We tend to assume that the IEC and the supervisors have considered all of the issues in the design and approval of the study. However, we really need to protect research participants *and* researchers by setting minimum standards for research training and supervision.

Geraldine Lee-Treweek and Stephanie Linkogle (2000a:15) highlight that 'unlike a social worker or qualified counsellor, a researcher is rarely trained in such issues as managing distress, ending difficult interactions and identifying ways in which a person could be helped or encouraged to help themselves'. Other authors have suggested carrying mobile phones (Bloor *et al.*, 2007; Langford, 2000; Liamputtong, 2007) and reporting back to supervisors at the conclusion of an interview as a way to enhance researcher safety.

One organization currently working towards ensuring the safety of all researchers is the Social Research Association (SRA) based in the United Kingdom. The SRA has developed *a Code of Practice for the Safety of Social Researchers*, which is designed for use by 'research funders, employers, research managers and researchers carrying out fieldwork'(Social Research Association, 2006). The guidelines focus on ensuring the safety (both physical and psychological) of social researchers. The code specifically examines some of the risks that social researchers may be confronted with when they are involved in research. The following risks (see Box 6.2) have been identified by the SRA as worthy of consideration by researchers.

The code is designed to alert all those involved in research to the safety issues that need to be considered in both the design and conduct of social

---

Box 6.2 Risks to be considered by researchers involved in sensitive research

- Risk of physical threat or abuse
- Risk of psychological trauma, as a result of actual or threatened violence or the nature of what is disclosed during the interaction
- Risk of being in a compromising situation, in which there might be accusations of improper behaviour
- Increased exposure to the risks of everyday life and social interaction, such as road accidents and infectious illness
- Risk of causing psychological harm or physical harm to others.

Box 6.3 Safety issues for consideration by researchers

- Clarifying responsibilities
- Budgeting for safety
- Planning for safety in research design
- Assessing risk in the fieldwork site
- Risk and respondents
- Setting up fieldwork
- Interview precautions
- Maintaining contact
- Conduct of interview
- Strategies for handling risk situations
- Debriefing and support after the event
- Making guidelines stick.

research. The main topics covered in the code of practice have been summarized in Box 6.3.

Reiterated throughout the code is the concept of the 'duty of care' that employers have to employees and it points out that 'safety at work is a dual responsibility of the employer and the employee' (Social Research Association, 2006:4), which highlights that safety is not the responsibility of the researcher alone. The main aim of this document focuses around risk reduction and includes all aspects of research including budgets and planning. It states that 'project costs might include extra fieldwork time (working in pairs, providing a 'shadow' or reporting back to base), taxis or hired cars, appropriate overnight accommodation, special training and counselling for staff researching sensitive topics' (p. 2).

A qualitative methods group (Qualti) based at Cardiff University in Wales, funded by the Economic and Social Research Council National Centre (ESRC) has recently published *A Commissioned Inquiry into the Risk to Well-Being of Researchers in Qualitative Research* (Bloor *et al.*, 2007). This inquiry began in 2006 and was undertaken to identify the risks that researchers face in their day-to-day work. The findings of the inquiry confirmed that many researchers face issues related to physical risks, gender and risk, emotional risk and institutional risk management.

Risk assessment and occupational health and safety

Like many Western countries, in Australia all workers are covered by the Occupational Health and Safety Act (Comcare, 1991). Under this legislation all workplaces are mandated to 'do as much as is reasonably practicable to protect the health and safety of employees at work' (Comcare, 1991:2). Like the SRA code, such legislation and related documents seek to remind employers that they must extend their definitions of safety beyond physical safety to also include psychological safety.

Researchers need to be aware that they are employees of institutions and therefore 'the risks they face can be considered within the framework of employment legislation designed to protect all workers' (Lee-Treweek & Linkogle, 2000a:197). As discussed above, the guidelines outlined in the SRA's code also seek to remind research institutes and universities about their obligations surrounding health and safety legislation to ensure that the potential for harm to researchers is minimized.

As we have presented earlier in this book, research work can be emotionally draining and exhausting and it may lead to researcher burn-out (Dickson-Swift *et al.*, 2007). While it has been argued that psychological injury may be caused by problems outside of the work environment, the Australian Safety Rehabilitation Act (1988) states that it is only necessary for work to make a 'material contribution' to the psychological injury to make it compensatable (Comcare, 2003:3). Based on this it is possible that researchers suffering such ill effects from their research may be eligible to claim compensation from their employer. Most universities and research institutes are aware of their legal responsibilities to their workers, which would include postgraduate research students. Universities and research centres are also covered by insurance policies that provide cover for harm experienced by employees and students during their employment or studies. We are required to undertake a risk assessment if we want to take a group of students on a field trip and provide formal risk assessment documentation to the university; however, the same does not apply to all research students' fieldwork. There are some disciplines that require formal risk assessments for student researchers (e.g. natural sciences) but despite the numerous guidelines and documentation of risks to researchers, the adoption of formal guidelines for qualitative researchers has yet to be widely adopted by the research community.

Department heads may be wrongly assuming that grant-holders or supervisors have undertaken the necessary risk assessments when they have not, which may put the university in an awkward position with the insurers should any researcher be harmed in the process of carrying out research. Many of the risk assessment forms currently used in academic institutions focus narrowly on physical risks; however, as we have outlined in this chapter, there is potential for both physical and emotional harm to take place.

Funding bodies also have a role to play in ensuring that this type of research is properly risk assessed (Bloor *et al.*, 2007). While it has been argued that funding bodies only have a minor role in researcher safety, because they contract out the research to be done on their behalf, some formalized procedures outlining their responsibilities would be advantageous (Bloor et al., 2007). Further discussion of the roles and responsibilities of research funders and supervisors is presented in Chapter 7.

Training, supervision and skill requirements

The researchers that we interviewed were asked to comment on the types of training that they thought might be useful for researchers undertaking this type of research. Many of their responses focused on the skills needed to talk with people who are often in very vulnerable situations highlighting that the provision of training for new researchers was important.

What I would like to see in the future is for research that is being undertaken in sensitive areas – that there be some, some sort of instruction, or guidelines, somewhere where it says things like 'now do you realise that when you are doing this sort of research, that these are issues that may come up for you?'. . . I think it would be important for that sort of thing to be raised in postgraduate seminars or written into some sort of research training.

I guess that anybody who is doing research in the human laboratory ought to be aware of the implications of people conducting research with people and on people and I think, that to me that is something that ought to be in every postgrad handbook, when they give you the guidelines and that sort of thing there should be something I think on that for people to reflect on.

I think that you do need some training 'cause you are going into some remote areas of people's psyches . . . that is not an easy thing to do, what happens if you get in there and stuff up that person's head . . . you need to know how to get out, some skills, definitely.

A number of the researchers we interviewed also felt that specific training in counselling skills were needed for researchers involved in research on sensitive topics.

I had some previous counselling skills training. I had come from a health background but I don't think that the counselling that you learn as part of a health course is adequate but yes certainly having been specifically trained in counselling skills would have been great.

I'm not a practitioner as such but I have done some counselling in the jobs that I have had. I was a Lifeline [crisis] telephone counsellor and I've done counselling at various other times in my professional career – and I think that did help – significantly.

I think that counselling skills would be helpful in terms of . . . even just knowing what to say.

While a number of the researchers did have training in counselling skills, or were qualified counsellors, others felt that possessing these types of skills may hinder the research and create boundary problems between research and service delivery.

Having a counselling background was difficult for me; I found it hard not to swap over to a counselling role and offer support and advice.

Some researchers we interviewed reported carrying mobile (cell) phones and reporting back to supervisors as strategies used to minimize the physical risks to themselves while conducting research.

I always have a phone and I tell someone where I will be and what time I expect to be back, that's just commonsense.

When I have finished an interview I call my supervisor so that she knows I am back safely.

However, it appears that strategies for risk reduction used by the researchers interviewed were not based on formal guidelines but were made on an ad hoc basis with supervisors. Although some researchers were aware of the risks to their physical safety there were others who reported finding themselves in risky situations without any prior consideration of the risks.

Sometimes it's a bit scary, I remember one interview I did, I drove for what seemed like ages up to this farm house, I had never met this man before and here I was in the middle of nowhere, asking a stranger questions about HIV infection. I didn't have a phone, I was being really careful, so no-one really knew where I was.

I had never met this person before; he'd been recruited over the phone, sounded like a nice guy so I went to his place for the interview. When I got there he asked to be interviewed in the bedroom because there were other people in the house. So I went in and he had laid out a mirror and all these massage oils and he kept saying 'look I've got these really lovely massage oils'. . . I was really upset when I left – I mean nothing happened but it really destabilized me because this was my first interview on the project. These kinds of dangers are distinctly possible.

In order to deal with some of these risks it has been suggested that researchers should be encouraged to seek supervision outside of the university setting (Brannen, 1988; Corden, Sainsbury, Sloper *et al.*, 2005; Coyle, 1998; Etherington, 1996; Hubbard *et al.*, 2001; Wray *et al.*, 2007). Kim Etherington (1996:346) suggests that 'as counsellors, we take this for granted; as researchers it is equally important'. Some researchers we interviewed reported using formalized support like supervision and debriefing outside of the university setting.

I do what psychologists do and they pay for supervision, so I pay for a supervisor outside the university and someone that is very skilled at working through these kinds of issues, like counselling issues as I see them so I would actually – quite separate to the university system that doesn't quite understand . . . I mean it's grappling with lots of issues around qualitative research and one thing it doesn't understand is the emotional content of it. So these days . . . it's that . . . Because if you don't actually process it you just carry it and that's detrimental to yourself.

There is now growing acceptance among qualitative researchers that there is a possibility that researchers involved in research on a sensitive topic may need some therapeutic support to deal with issues that may arise from the research. Potential emotional risks for researchers may include such things as identification with people who have bad experiences or pain, which may then go on to produce feelings of sadness, anger or depression in researchers (Kleinman & Copp, 1993). Published accounts of researchers being affected by their work on sensitive topics include Linda Dunn's (1991) account of believing that interviewing women who had suffered abuse led to her own serious sleep disorders and psychosomatic complaints requiring medication and therapy, and Hilary Davis' (2001) description of the impact of observing death and intensive care in a public hospital setting and how she needed to talk through her experiences. Natalie Wray and colleagues (2007), in their study of gynaecological cancers, reported using both the university counsellor for debriefing after emotionally distressing interviews and utilizing a fee-for-service psychotherapist to assist in dealing with distress. Accounts like these led a group of researchers working in the Social Policy Research Unit (SPRU) at the University of York to consider how best to manage emotional risks in research for their researchers. This team decided to explore the possibility of some professional support to assist them manage feelings that might be evoked as a result of undertaking research with bereaved parents (Corden *et al.*, 2005). The SPRU team used a model of group psychotherapy that provided a safe space for reflection and to assist researchers to develop awareness of their own feelings around loss.

In addition to counselling and support, reflexive journaling and working in teams have successfully been used by researchers in order to ameliorate some of the difficulties associated with researching sensitive topics (Malacrida, 2007). Claudia Malacrida (2007) provides an account of the benefits of using such an approach in her study regarding mothering when disabled. The journaling initially stemmed from her concern about the well-being of the researchers working on the project; however, it went on to provide an account of the issues faced by the researchers involved in the 'emotionally laden' research. She highlights that while self-reflexive journaling is relatively common in the curriculum for professional and personal development in professional training for family therapy, nursing and social work students (Darlington & Scott, 2002; Lee, Eppler, Kendal *et al.*, 2001; Ruthman *et al.*, 2004; Tillman, 2003), it should also be considered for researchers due to the emotional nature of sensitive research. Journaling should begin early in the research and can provide safe opportunities for researchers, research assistants and transcribers to engage in written reflection on the research process.

As we have previously outlined, universities (and research centres) have a duty of care to researchers (and participants) to ensure that they are not harmed in any way (physically or emotionally) from their participation in research and making provisions for support like this ensures that the duty of care is followed.

Most postgraduate students have access to regular supervision within the university setting from their immediate supervisors. However, other more experienced researchers attached to universities or large research centres may not necessarily have access to regular formalized supervision. Although accessing support from outside of the university setting may assist researchers in dealing with issues that arise from their participation in research, feelings of guilt have been reported by researchers who utilize such support stating that accessing support can feel a little 'self indulgent' (Corden *et al.*, 2005:157). Researchers may feel a sense of guilt for using funds available for the research to pay for regular supervision.

It is important for researchers working on sensitive topics to have strategies in place that give them the opportunity to talk about their research experiences. With a lack of formalized support mechanisms some researchers have reported using less formal arrangements. For example, debriefing can often take the form of an informal chat in the staff room or at the photocopier with colleagues (Hubbard *et al.*, 2001). It has also been reported that informal supervision and debriefing sessions are often provided by colleagues, friends and family members. Mick Bloor and colleagues (2007:34) sum up the problems associated with this.

Whilst it is inevitable to a certain extent that there will be off-loading at home, the formal exploitation of informal networks – for example, building them into research designs – is not deemed appropriate, and such strategies do not absolve research funders and institutions of their responsibilities to researchers.

One of the researchers we interviewed spoke of his own experiences with debriefing:

Look after yourself – have someone who you can debrief with, in fact have two people who you can debrief with. I would say, you are probably better off having someone who is a very close friend, well maybe it's good to have two – one who is a close friend and one who isn't so that you have the opportunity to do both.

Although many of the researchers interviewed espoused the benefits of debriefing and supervision, it is important to note that while these may be of benefit to some researchers, they may not necessarily suit everyone.

Summary

In this chapter we have discussed many of the inherent risks associated with undertaking research on sensitive topics. An overview of risk theory and how it applies to the actual conduct of research has been presented. We have discussed ethical issues including informed consent and confidentiality and have presented a range of suggestions for training and supervision to assist researchers to manage those risks. While we do not wish to be alarmist and suggest that undertaking sensitive research is not worth the effort, we do wish to draw readers' attention to the many risks and challenges that this type of research poses for researchers so that they can undertake a full assessment and ensure that they (and their participants) are not harmed (physically or emotionally) by research participation. In the following chapter we provide further elaboration on these points and provide some recommendations for researchers.

Tutorial activities

(a) In this chapter we discussed the importance of maintaining confidentially and anonymity. Consider the following scenario: you are undertaking a study that aims to document the experiences of HIV positive young gay men living in a rural town. What strategies can you put in place to ensure you protect the confidentiality of the research participants?

(b) We also discussed informed consent in the chapter. Consider the following scenario. You are undertaking a study that aims to explore the experiences of illiterate street kids. What strategies can you put in place to ensure that the consent to participate that you receive is truly informed?

(c) In this chapter we discussed the importance of assessing risk and the role of various key stakeholders in the research process. Access the application form for ethics approval for your institution. Does the form provide a space for you to reflect and assess risks for the researcher? Does the form (or the corresponding instructions) prompt you to consider risks to researchers? Are the risks considered both physical and psychological?

SUGGESTED READING

Christian, C.G. (2005). Ethics and politics in qualitative research. In N.K. Denzin & Y.S. Lincoln (eds.), *The Sage Handbook of Qualitative Research* (pp. 109–164). Thousand Oaks, CA: Sage Publications.

Dickson-Swift, V., James, E. & Kippen, S. (2005). Do university ethics committees adequately protect public health researchers? *Australian and New Zealand Journal of Public Health*, **29**(6), 576–582.

Lee-Treweek, G. & Linkogle, S. (eds.) (2000). *Danger in the Field: Risk and Ethics in Social Research*. London: Routledge.

Richards, H.M. & Schwartz, L.J. (2002). Ethics of qualitative research: are there special issues for health services research? *Family Practice*, **19**(2), 135–139.

Rosenblatt, P.C. (1995). Ethics of qualitative interviewing with grieving families. *Death Studies*, **19**, 139–155.

7

Implications and recommendations for researchers

In taking better care of the researchers, we might enhance the quality of the whole process, for the benefit of researched, researchers and the learning community alike.

(Etherington, 1996:346)

So, by this stage of the book readers may well be feeling like conducting research on a sensitive topic is fraught with problems and challenges and you might be rethinking your proposal! Do not despair. In this chapter we provide a number of practical recommendations to help reduce both the chance of negative outcomes and the impact they may have on you as a researcher. The aim of the earlier chapters was not to be alarmist, but instead to raise awareness of potential risks so as to minimize exposure of future researchers.

The factors that contribute to the risks described throughout this book are complex, and as such the solutions we suggest are multilevel and span responsibility from the individual researcher, the supervisor, the research institution and extend as far as granting bodies who fund research. Therefore, the recommendations we make are tailored for specific groups in the research process. While few readers are likely to be in a position to influence the activities and policies of their institution and national funding bodies, most of us do have the potential, and some would argue the responsibility, to try and influence our own research groups and our own individual behaviour.

The recommendations we discuss in this chapter are based on an international review of current best practice and also on the advice of researchers who have conducted sensitive research. In particular, we report the responses to a specific question: 'If you had to give advice to someone about to undertake research on a sensitive topic, what would you tell them?' So in a sense, this chapter is inviting you to sit in on our many conversations with both experienced and inexperienced researchers as they share their stories and wisdom. We believe that adoption of these recommendations will ensure that qualitative research on sensitive topics can continue to be conducted without adversely affecting those who are involved in it and we challenge readers to reflect on the recommendations made in this chapter, adopt those that are most relevant and continue on the exciting path of conducting research on sensitive topics.

Recommendations for individual researchers

While many readers may not be in a position to influence the policy and practice of their research institution or national funding bodies, there are many steps that you *can* take to protect yourself from both the physical and psychological risks associated with conducting sensitive research. This section describes the development of a comprehensive safety protocol that will allow you to consider a range of different strategies in a systematic way in discussion with your academic supervisor or research team leader. Barbara Paterson and colleagues (1999) provide a detailed description of the development of a safety protocol for researchers, with particular focus on protection from physical harm. This section is based heavily on their recommendations. However, we apply the process they describe to the protection of emotional and psychological harm rather than physical harm.

What is a safety protocol for researchers?

A safety protocol for researchers is intended to detail the policies and procedures for prevention, intervention and follow-up of harmful incidents encountered by researchers in the field. Traditionally, harmful events include physical and/or verbal aggression in which the physical and/or psychological safety of the researcher is jeopardized (Greater Vancouver Mental Health Service, 1996) and we expand this definition to include the potential emotional and psychological harm that can come from conducting face-to-face interviews with participants on a sensitive topic. As it may be easier for some readers to relate to issues of physical safety, for each consideration we include an example related to physical safety as well as examples relating to emotional and/or psychological safety.

Perhaps the best prevention of harm during fieldwork is the readiness of researchers to anticipate and mediate danger (Hayes, Carter, Carroll *et al.*, 1996). So, we recommend that research teams discuss and teach the management of danger in advance of data collection in the field and develop a safety protocol that is applicable to the research team's unique needs and situation. One good way to develop a safety protocol for research is to pose common dangerous situations (e.g. the researcher is required to use a stairwell in an apartment building to reach the participant's apartment on the third floor, and there are two people on the stairwell who watch the researcher in what appears to be a menacing way) and use these hypothetical situations to stimulate discussion in the research team about the most effective ways to respond to such a situation (Hayes *et al.*, 1996). In the case of sensitive qualitative research, the potential dangerous situations relate not only to physical safety, but also to emotional and psychological safety. For example, Jo Moran Ellis (1996:181), describes the emotional strain of having to deal with distressing situations or stories as 'pain by proxy' recounting how repeatedly listening to stories of child sexual abuse emotionally affected her.

In order to develop the safety protocol it is important to firstly identify potential risks, then identify possible prevention strategies and finally to document the research team's responsibilities and response in the prevention and management of the risks identified. Table 7.1 outlines some potential scenarios that may be applicable for consideration at the risk identification stage of the safety protocol development. We suggest that researchers work with their research team and/or supervisor to devise and discuss such scenarios.

The next step in the development of the safety protocol is devising potential preventive strategies. Box 7.1 lists a range of prevention strategies for researchers conducting sensitive qualitative research that may be worth considering in this phase of the development of the safety protocol.

The final step in devising the safety protocol is to document the research team's responsibilities and response in the prevention and management of the risks identified. For example, if a fieldworker fails to call in to report an interview is complete, what is the next step (inform the police?) and who is responsible for monitoring who has called in and who has not? We suggest that the various responsibilities are documented in writing and copies are shared within the research team and also form part of the application for research ethics approval.

Recommendations for those transcribing interviews

In qualitative research, many researchers choose to undertake their own transcription; however, some researchers do opt to have the transcription completed by another person outside of the fieldwork team. Transcribing data from a sensitive research interview has the potential to impact on the emotional health of the transcriber in the same way it can impact on the interviewer during fieldwork (Etherington, 2007; Gregory *et al.*, 1997; McCosker *et al.*, 2001; Wray *et al.*, 2007). The impact of the emotion may be exacerbated if the transcriber is also the one who collected the data in the first place, effectively requiring a re-living of the data. Based on this we recommend the adoption of the guidelines outlined in Box 7.2 as suggested by David Gregory, Cynthia Russell and Linda Phillips (1997).

Adoption of these guidelines will help ensure that transcribers are not harmed in the process of undertaking interview transcription.

Table 7.1. A framework for assessing the situation prior to beginning fieldwork in order to develop a safety protocol

Topics for consideration	Example relating to physical safety	Possible solution	Example relating to emotional and/or psychological safety	Possible solution
The research participants. Although qualitative researchers may face safety issues at any research interview, they are particularly vulnerable when studying certain types of participants.	Those with a known history of aggression, persons with dementia who are violent.	Interviews are conducted in a neutral setting such as a coffee shop or local community health centre rather than the home of the participant. Is an ethnically-matched interviewer a more appropriate choice?	Those who are experiencing or relating a personally traumatic event or episode, those who may be palliative, rape victims.	Spacing of interviews to reduce risk of emotional exhaustion.
The nature of the topic. Some research topics are associated with a higher degree of risk to the researcher than others.	Interviewing potentially aggressive and volatile participants about politically or emotionally charged topics, for example poverty, unemployment, marital breakdown.	The researcher should be accompanied in the field by another member of the research team. Utilize mobile phones, provide your itinerary to a research supervisor and report back when finished.	The topic of research has potential to raise unresolved issues for the researcher, for example miscarriage, grief over the loss of a loved one.	Reflect on how the researcher became interested in the topic and the likelihood that the interviews may bring up unresolved issues. Reflect on the likelihood of vicarious traumatization. Instigate informal peer support and formalized supervision to allow for debriefing and personal reflection.

Nature of the environment. The location of the setting of data collection is significant in researcher safety.	Conducting fieldwork in transient, single-room neighbourhoods where drug use and criminal activity are common.	The researcher and a companion drive to the area on a day prior to conducting the research to assess the safety of the surroundings, including the existence of well-lit, accessible parking spaces, and to check the accuracy of directions to the street and building to avoid being lost or wandering without an escort in an unfamiliar neighbourhood. (See SRA code for further suggestions.)
	Conducting a series of interviews in the home of a participant may contribute to a blurring of boundaries between researcher and friend.	Discuss and plan strategies regarding level of personal disclosure, strategies to end the relationship, levels of contact outside of the research relationship.

Box 7.1 Prevention strategies for researchers conducting sensitive qualitative research

1. **Utilize informal networks** of friends and family to allow opportunities for debriefing.
2. **Formalize arrangement in a peer support programme** that brings together a range of researchers involved in similar research for group sessions. This may include some form of researcher support to improve psychological well-being in the form of a professional confidante (Brannen, 1988; Johnson & Clarke, 2003; Kitson *et al.*, 1996; Stoler, 2002).
3. **Organize access to professional supervision** (Ferguson, 2003; Kitson *et al.*, 1996; Payne, 1994; Ridge, Hee & Aroni, 1999; Wray, Markovic & Manderson, 2007) to provide opportunities for self-development and self-care, and to strengthen the process of self-reflection and self-monitoring (McMahon & Patton, 2002). Researchers could potentially use supervision sessions for debriefing, mentoring and skill development, all of which will enhance a researcher's ability to undertake research without damaging their health and well-being. Access to professional supervision (which may be outside of the university) may assist researchers to deal with the potential stress associated with undertaking research and avoid burn-out.
4. **Consider strategies for emotional distancing** if the research topic or participants are likely to lead to emotion work on the part of the researcher (see Chapter 5).
5. **Prior to fieldwork beginning**, plan how you will approach:
   • rapport development
   • levels of self-disclosure
   • physical displays of emotion during the interview
   • strategies to end the relationship.
6. **Reflect on how you became interested in the topic** of the research and whether the interviews are likely to raise unresolved issues for you (see Chapter 6). Keep a reflexive research journal documenting the issues you face throughout the research.
7. **Consider the potential for vicarious traumatization** depending upon the topic of the interviews (see Chapter 6).
8. **Timetable interviews to allow sufficient recovery time** to reduce the risk of emotional exhaustion and to allow time for reflection on the physical and emotional aspects of research (see Chapter 6).
9. **Become familiar with the signs of burn-out** and instigate a system to identify burn-out symptoms early should they occur.
10. **Instigate strategies to promote self-care** to minimize the harm you may be exposed to as part of your research work (Brannen, 1988; Campbell, 2002; James & Platzer, 1999; Rager, 2005a; Renzetti & Lee, 1993; Rowling, 1999).

Box 7.2 Recommendations to protect the emotional safety
of transcribers

1. Be included in the ethical clearance process.
2. Be informed of the nature of the research and the type of data.
3. Be alerted prior to the transcription of potentially 'challenging' or
   'difficult' interviews.
4. Have regular scheduled debriefing sessions.
5. Have prompt access to an appropriate person for crisis counselling.
6. Have a clearly documented termination from the transcription process,
   that includes a resolution of personal issues that arose as a consequence
   of the work.
7. Be encouraged to journal thoughts and feelings, which may then become
   part of the fieldwork notes in some research approaches.

(*Source:* Gregory, Russell & Phillips, 1997)

Recommendations for those supervising research (chief investigators/research leaders)

Supervisors, research leaders and chief investigators (CIs) clearly have responsibilities to the researchers they manage, and the supervisor needs to take responsibility for risk assessment for the researchers involved in their projects. Chief investigators need to actively create an atmosphere where researchers feel comfortable in sharing their concerns about the research. This should not focus too narrowly on just the research process: that is, how the interviews went, how the questions flowed, or the nature of the data obtained. It should, rather, aim to create an environment where researchers feel able to talk openly about issues that the research may have raised for them. Chief investigators have an important role to play in debriefing researchers who may or may not have been emotionally affected by their research. However, if the CI is unable to provide appropriate and timely debriefing they should actively seek an alternative arrangement for the researcher/interviewer. It is important to note that some researchers may choose not to use their CI for this role, fearing that they may be judged incompetent, and therefore researchers should be given the option to use independent supervision.

Chief investigators are in an ideal situation to ensure that researchers are aware of the difficulties they may face throughout the research. They need to ensure that the researchers (including transcribers and research assistants) have the necessary skills and training they need to undertake the research. This may require a skills audit by the CI prior to the commencement of fieldwork. Chief investigators should encourage researchers to undertake

> **Box 7.3** Recommendations for research supervisors to protect research staff from psychological and emotional harm
>
> 1. Initiate and drive processes to **develop safety protocols** to protect members of your research team (including fieldworkers, transcribers).
> 2. **Create an environment** where researchers feel able to talk openly about challenging issues.
> 3. Carry out a **skills audit** of your fieldwork staff prior to employment on projects exploring sensitive topics.
> 4. Provide **professional supervision** and opportunities for interviewers and transcribers to debrief and reflect on the interview process. This can be either directly or via funding and negotiating external supervision opportunities.
> 5. **Incorporate discussions of psychological well-being** and emotional risk into professional development seminars and research coursework.
>
> (*Source:* Social Research Association, 2006)

planning for their own physical and emotional safety including the development of protocols for researcher safety. There may also be potential for a structured mentoring programme to be developed for novice researchers involved in sensitive projects to ensure that they are provided with support in a timely and ongoing fashion.

Chief investigators need to actively seek out opportunities to openly discuss the issues faced by researchers. This could take the form of a series of seminars for both new and experienced researchers addressing some of the challenges they may face. This will create a space within academia for the open discussion of the issues for researchers, thus normalizing discussions on issues such as managing emotions, boundary blurring and avoiding burn-out. Box 7.3 summarizes the recommendations for research supervisors designed to protect research staff from psychological and emotional harm.

Recommendations for research institutions

As discussed in Chapter 6, there are a number of issues that need to be addressed at the institutional level. Institutional ethics committees (IECs) need to be made explicitly aware of the potential risks faced by *researchers* undertaking social research, especially on sensitive topics. They need to factor these risks into their assessment of the ethical issues in research that they review, and not just focus on risks to research participants. In Australia, the body overseeing IECs has recently amended its guidelines to incorporate

Box 7.4 Relevant guidelines for IECs in Australia

1. Qualitative research that explores sensitive topics in depth may involve emotional and other risks to both participant and researcher. There should be clear protocols for dealing with distress that might be experienced by participants.
2. Predicting what topics are likely to lead to distress will not always be easy. Researchers should have sufficient training to help them in making such predictions.
3. Qualitative research may involve methods of data collection that require the development of personal relationships with participants. Researchers should reflect on the impact that they may have on the participants and vice versa, and as far as possible should describe in the research proposal any anticipated impact of this nature.

(*Source:* NHMRC, 2007)

risks to qualitative researchers, thereby requiring that IECs in Australia extend their responsibilities beyond ensuring the safety of research subjects and include researchers in their assessments of risk (NHMRC, 2007). The recent amendments are outlined in Box 7.4.

The NHMRC (1995, 2007) asks IECs to ensure that the researchers have a sufficient skill base to carry out the research. However, an explanation of exactly what skills might be required has not been provided. It is currently very difficult for IEC members to make judgements regarding the researcher's skill level as this information is not explicitly requested by most IECs (Dickson-Swift *et al.*, 2005) and there are no minimum standards set. The NHMRC (and similar bodies internationally) have a role to play in developing guidelines for researchers and IECs so that they can be satisfied that researchers are not undertaking research that may be damaging to their physical and/ or psychological well-being. This is supported by the recent commissioned report titled *Risk to Well-Being of Researchers in Qualitative Research* that concluded that all university ethics committees should accept formal responsibility for oversight of provision for postgraduate student safety, with safety issues being addressed in the context of a specific question on the application form and of the guidance notes on form completion (Bloor *et al.*, 2007).

Research institutions need to be aware of the issues that research into sensitive topics may raise for the researchers and to have in place some strategies to help researchers to deal with those issues. This should not be done on an ad hoc basis, but instead needs to be written into the policies (such as occupational health and safety, and ethics) that govern research practice. The ethics approval process should include a section examining how the researcher proposes to handle the issues of self-disclosure, leaving the relationship, boundary blurring and researcher self-care, and what impact the proposed research may have on transcribers. While qualitative studies of sensitive topics may place the researcher in situations of particular personal risk, all research that entails any direct contact with the public presents a potential risk. Researchers and research institutions should develop and maintain awareness of such risks to themselves and their colleagues and make every effort to diminish the dangers.

There is, therefore, a need for institutional level research policies. Such policies should include formal guidelines (perhaps as checklists for researchers to go through prior to beginning the research and periodic health and safety audits of departments that include provision for content on researcher safety) (Bloor *et al.*, 2007) and should also address the minimum level of training and support needed for undertaking sensitive research. Guidelines for researchers have been successfully adopted by social researchers in the United Kingdom (see Chapter 6; SRA code of practice), which provide an excellent starting point for a set of guidelines to be developed for use by institutions that contain qualitative researchers involved in sensitive research. These guidelines could identify both physical and psychological safety issues that need to be considered when designing and conducting sensitive research and encourage risk reduction for researchers, and could cover issues such as clarifying responsibilities, budgeting, planning for safety in research design, assessing risks and strategies for handling risks.

Recommendations for funding bodies

The granting bodies that provide funding for research need to be aware of the issues that involvement in sensitive research can raise for researchers. Gill Hubbard and colleagues (2001) discuss the role of the granting bodies in the acknowledgement of the emotional dimension of this type of research. They call for the establishment of a 'responsive and supportive culture, which acknowledges upfront that researchers may experience emotions during and after fieldwork' (Hubbard *et al.*, 2001:134). Granting bodies must openly encourage researchers to factor in the additional costs that may be incurred in the conduct of sensitive research (such as additional fieldwork time to allow working in pairs, providing a 'shadow' or reporting back to base, taxis or hire cars, appropriate overnight accommodation, special training, counselling for staff; SRA code of practice). A failure to provide a researcher with the necessary support could have an impact on both the success of the project and the health and well-being of the researcher. The emotional impact that the research can have on the researchers is an issue that:

research funding agencies and research managers must take into account if they are not to compromise the health of fieldworkers. In particular, funding agencies need to take into account the stresses involved in such research and must be prepared, not only for such research to take time, but also to ensure that research teams are adequately staffed to allow fieldworkers space for 'remissions – i.e. periods away from the field – and 'reminders' – time to do other things (teach, write) – which might allow them to gain some psychological distance from the stresses involved. (Melrose, 2002:349)

Risk to Well-Being of Researchers in Qualitative Research recommends that all funders should require principle investigators to comply with the SRA guidelines for researcher safety, and that they should invite referees to comment on researcher safety issues as part of the assessment of applicants' research methods (Bloor *et al.*, 2007; Social Research Association, 2006). We strongly support these recommendations.

Summary

The importance of continuing high-quality qualitative research on sensitive topics is paramount to the success of health and social sciences research into the future. Researchers need to continually push the boundaries of research methodologies, finding new ways to undertake research on the growing list of health and social issues faced by society. The growth of qualitative research in health and well-being is testimony to our need to explore and document the many issues faced by a complex society that have direct and indirect impacts on health. A number of recommendations for safe practice have been made. If instigated, these recommendations should ensure that qualitative research on sensitive topics can be conducted in a way that appropriately protects the researchers involved.

The aim of this book was to document the experiences of a range of health and social science researchers undertaking qualitative research on sensitive topics and to present some recommendations for researchers to consider when planning a project. While the researchers whose stories we retell here were all working broadly in sensitive areas, their experiences and the recommendations we make are applicable to *any* researcher who is embarking on a qualitative project. Qualitative research is a 'journey of discovery' that can be simultaneously challenging and inspiring in amazing and unforseen ways (Waldrop, 2004:236). We hope that we have assisted readers to recognize some of those ethical, practical and methodological challenges that are inherent in researching sensitive topics and that readers continue to be inspired to undertake such research well into the future. We wish you well with your research.

Tutorial activities

(a) In this chapter we discussed the importance of developing a safety protocol prior to beginning fieldwork. Devise a hypothetical research project and create some potential scenarios as part of the development of a safety protocol for the project.

(b) Draw up a list of practical strategies that could be used to protect transcribers working on interview data from survivors of childhood abuse and neglect.

SUGGESTED READING

Bloor, M., Fincham, B. & Sampson, H. (2007). *Qualti (NCRM) Commissioned Inquiry into the Risk to Well-Being of Researchers in Qualitative Research*. Cardiff: Cardiff ESRC National Centre for Research Methods, Cardiff University.

Paterson, B.L., Gregory, D. & Thorne, S. (1999). A protocol for researcher safety. *Qualitative Health Research*, **9**(2), 259–269.

Social Research Association (2006). *A Code of Practice for the Safety of Social Researchers*. Available at: www.the-sra.org.uk/ [Accessed 31/3/2008].

References

Acker, J., Barry, K. & Essevald, J. (1991). Objectivity and truth: problems in doing feminist research. In M.M. Fonow & J.A. Cook (eds.), *Beyond Methodology: Feminist Scholarship as Lived Research* (pp.133–153). Bloomington: Indianna University Press.

Aldridge, M. (1994). Unlimited liability? Emotional labour in nursing and social work. *Journal of Advanced Nursing*, **20**, 722–728.

Alexander, J.G., de Chesnay, M., Marshall, E. *et al.* (1989). Parallel reactions in rape victims and rape researchers. *Violence and Victims*, **4**(1), 57–62.

Allan, H. (2006). Using participant observation to immerse onself in the field: the relevance and importance of ethnography for illuminating the role of emotions in nursing practice. *Journal of Research in Nursing*, **11**(5), 397–407.

Allen, K.R. & Walker, A.J. (1992). A feminist analysis of interviews with elderly mothers and their daughters. In J.F. Gilgun, K. Daly & G. Handel (eds.), *Qualitative Methods in Family Research* (pp.198–214). Newbury Park, CA: Sage Publications.

Alty, A. & Rodham, K. (1998). The ouch! factor: problems in conducting sensitive research. *Qualitative Health Research*, **8**(2), 275–282.

Ashforth, B. & Humphrey, R.H. (1993). Emotional labour in service roles: the influence of identity. *Academy of Management Review*, **18**, 88–115.

Atkinson, P., Coffey, A. & Delamont, S. (2003). *Key Themes in Qualitative Research: Continuities and Change.* New York: AltaMira Press.

Australian Association of Social Workers (1999). *AASW Code of Ethics.* Canberra: Australian Association of Social Workers.

Australian Guidance and Counselling Association (1997). *Code of Ethics.* Canberra: Australian Guidance and Counselling Association.

Australian Nursing Council (2003) *Code of Conduct for Nurses in Australia.* Canberra: Australian Nursing Council.

Australian Psychological Society (2002). *Code of Ethics.* Melbourne: Australian Psychological Society.

Baker, L., Lavende, T. & Tincello, D. (2005). Factors that influence women's decisions about whether to participate in research: an exploratory study. *Birth*, **32**(1), 60–66.

Barnard, M. (2005). Discomforting research: colliding moralities and looking for 'truth' in a study of parental drug problems. *Sociology of Health and Illness*, **27**(1), 1–19.

Batchelor, J.A. & Briggs, C.A. (1994). Subject, project of self? Thoughts on ethical dilemmas for social and medical researchers. *Social Science and Medicine*, **39**(7), 949–954.

Beauchamp, T.L. & Childress, J.F. (1994). *Principles of Biomedical Ethics* (3rd edn). Oxford: Oxford University Press.

Beauchamp, T.L., Jennings, B., Kinney, E.D. & Levine, R.J. (2002). Pharmaceutical research involving the homeless. *Journal of Medicine and Philosophy,* **27**(5), 547–564.

Beaver, K., Luker, K. & Woods, S. (1999). Conducting research with the terminally ill: challenges and considerations. *International Journal of Palliative Nursing,* **5**(1), 13–18.

Beck, U. (1992). *Risk Society.* London: Sage Publications.

Beck, U. (1994). The reinvention of politics: towards a theory of reflexive modernization. In U. Beck, A. Giddens & S. Lash (eds.), *Reflexive Modernization: Politics, Traditions and Aesthetics in the Modern Social Order* (pp. 1–55). Cambridge: Polity Press.

Becker, H.S. (1963). *Outsiders: Studies in the Sociology of Deviance.* New York: Free Press.

Beehr, T.A. (1995). Role ambiguity and role conflict in the workplace. In T.A. Beehr (ed.), *Psychological Stress in the Workplace* (pp. 55–82). New York: Routledge.

Behar, R. (1996). *The Vulnerable Observer: Anthropology That Breaks Your Heart.* Boston: Beacon.

Bell, C. & Encel, S. (1978). *Inside the Whale: Ten Personal Accounts of Social Research.* Rushcutters Bay: Pergamon Press.

Bell, C. & Newby, H. (1977). *Doing Sociological Research.* London: Allen and Unwin.

Bellas, M.L. (1999). Emotional labor in academia: the case of professors. *Annals of the American Academy of Political and Social Science,* **561**, 91–110.

Bendelow, G. & Williams, S.J. (1998). Introduction: emotions in social life. Mapping the sociological terrain. In G. Bendelow & S.J. Williams (eds.), *Emotions in Social Life: Critical Themes and Contemporary Issues* (pp. xv–xxx). London: Routledge.

Benner, P. (2000). The roles of embodiment, emotion and rationality and agency in nursing practice. *Nursing Philosophy,* **1**, 5–19.

Bennett, O., Evans, R.G. & Tattersall, A. (1993). Stress and coping in social workers: a preliminary investigation. *British Journal of Social Work,* **23**, 31–44.

Bergen, R.K. (1993). Interviewing survivors of marital rape: doing feminist research on sensitive topics. In C. Renzetti & R.M. Lee (eds.), *Researching Sensitive Topics* (pp. 197–211). Newbury Park: Sage Publications.

Berk, R.A. & Adams, J.M. (2001). Establishing rapport with deviant groups. In J.M. Miller & R. Tewksbury (eds.), *Extreme Methods: Innovative Approaches to Social Science Research* (pp. 58–71). Boston: Allyn and Bacon.

Birch, M. & Miller, T. (2000). Inviting intimacy: the interview as therapeutic opportunity. *International Journal of Social Research Methodology,* **3**(3), 189–202.

Bloor, M., Fincham, B. & Sampson, H. (2007). *Qualti (NCRM) Commissioned Inquiry into the Risk to Well-Being of Researchers in Qualitative Research.* Cardiff: Cardiff ESRC National Centre for Research Methods, Cardiff University.

Booth, S. (1999). Researching health and homelessness: methodological challenges for researchers working with a vulnerable, hard-to-reach, transient population. *Australian Journal of Primary Health,* **5**(3), 76–81.

Booth, T. & Booth, W. (1994). The use of depth interviewing with vulnerable subjects. *Social Science and Medicine,* **39**(2), 415–424.

Bosk, C.L. (2002). Obtaining voluntary consent for research in desperately ill patients. *Medical Care,* **40**(9), Supplement V64–V68.

Bourdieu, P. (1988). *Homo academicus* (P. Collier, Trans.). Cambridge: Polity Press.

Bourdieu, P. & Wacquant, J.D. (1992). *Invitation to Reflexive Sociology*. Cambridge: Polity Press.

Brannen, J. (1988). The study of sensitive subjects. *The Sociological Review*, **36**, 552–563.

Brannen, J. (1993). The effects of research on participants: the findings from a study of mothers and employment. *The Sociological Review*, **41**(2), 328–346.

Brewer, J.D. (1993). Sensitivity as a problem in field research. In C.M. Renzetti & R.M. Lee (eds.), *Researching Sensitive Topics*. Newbury Park: Sage Publications.

Broom, A. & Willis, E. (2007). Competing paradigms and health research. In M. Saks & J. Allsop (eds.), *Researching Health: Qualitative, Quantitative and Mixed Methods* (pp.16–31). London: Sage Publications.

Bulmer, M. (1984). *The Chicago School of Sociology: Institutionalization, Diversity and the Rise of Sociological Research*. Chicago: Chicago University Press.

Burkitt, I. (1997). Social relationships and emotions. *Sociology*, **31**(1), 37–55.

Burr, G. (1995). Unfinished business: interviewing family members of critically ill patients. *Nursing Inquiry*, **3**, 172–177.

Calhoun, C., LiPuma, E. & Postone, M. (eds.) (1992). *Bourdieu: Critical Perspectives*. Cambridge: Polity Press.

Cameron, M. (1993). *Living with AIDS: Experiencing Ethical Problems*. Newbury Park: Sage Publications.

Campbell, R. (2002). *Emotionally Involved: The Impact of Researching Rape*. New York: Routledge.

Campbell, R. & Salem, D.A. (1999). Concept mapping as a feminist research method: examining the community response to rape. *Psychology of Women Quarterly*, **23**, 67–91.

Campbell, R. & Wasco, S.M. (2000). Feminist approaches to social science: epistemological and methodological tenets. *American Journal of Community Psychology*, **28**(6), 773–791.

Cannon, S. (1989). Social research in stressful settings: difficulties for the sociologist studying the treatment of breast cancer. *Sociology of Health and Illness*, **11**(1), 62–77.

Cannon, S. (1992). Reflections on fieldwork in stressful settings. In R.G. Burgess (ed.), *Studies in Qualitative Methodology* (Vol. 3). *Learning About Fieldwork* (pp.147–182). Greenwich: JAI Press.

Carter, K. & Delamont, S. (eds.) (1996). *Qualitative Research: The Emotional Dimension*. Aldershot: Avebury.

Cataldi, S. (1993). *Emotion, Depth, and Flesh: A Study of Sensitive Space. Reflections on Merleau-Ponty's Philosophy of Embodiment*. Albany: SUNY Press.

Ceglowski, D. (2000). Research as relationship. *Qualitative Inquiry*, **6**(1), 88–103.

Central Office for Research Ethics Committees (COREC) (2006). NHS Research Ethics Committee Application Form. Available from http://www.corec.org.uk/applicants/index.htm [Accessed 2/7/2006].

Charmaz, K. (1991). *Good Days, Bad Days: The Self in Chronic Illness and Time*. New Brunswick: Rutgers University Press.

Charmaz, K. (2000). Grounded theory: objectivist and constructivist methods. In N. Denzin & Y. Lincoln (eds.), *Handbook of Qualitative Research* (2nd edn, pp.509–535). Thousand Oaks, CA: Sage Publications.

Cherniss, C. (1995). *Beyond Burnout: Helping Teachers, Nurses, Therapists and Lawyers Recover from Stress and Disillusionment*. New York: Routledge.

Christian, C.G. (2005). Ethics and politics in qualitative research. In N.K. Denzin & Y.S. Lincoln (eds.), *The Sage Handbook of Qualitative Research* (3rd edn, pp. 109–164). Thousand Oaks, CA: Sage Publications.

Clifford, C. (1997). *Nursing and Healthcare Research: A Skills-based Introduction* (2nd edn). London: Prentice Hall.

Coffey, A. (1999). *The Ethnographic Self: Fieldwork and the Representation of Identity*. London: Sage Publications.

Comcare (1991). Occupational Health and Safety (Commonwealth Employment) Act. Available from http://www.comcare.gov.au/ohs/publications-index.html [Accessed 21/3/2004].

Comcare (2003). Preventing and Managing Psychological Injuries in the Workplace: Managers Guide. Available from http://www.comcare.gov.au/pdf-files/stress-agency.pdf [Accessed 20/4/2004].

Cook, A.S. & Bosley, G. (1995). The experience of participating in bereavement research: stressful or therapeutic? *Death Studies*, **19**, 157–170.

Copp, M. (1998). When emotion work is doomed to fail: ideological and structural constraints on emotion management. *Symbolic Interaction*, **21**, 299–328.

Corden, A., Sainsbury, R., Sloper, R. & Ward, B. (2005). Using a model of group psychotherapy to support social research on sensitive topics. *International Journal of Social Research Methodology*, **8**(2), 151–160.

Corey, G., Corey, M. & Callanan, P. (2003). *Issues and Ethics in the Helping Professions* (6th edn). Pacific Grove, CA: Brooks/Cole.

Cotterill, P. (1992). Interviewing women: issues of friendship, vulnerability and power. *Women's Studies International Forum*, **15**(5/6), 593–606.

Cowles, K.V. (1988). Issues in qualitative research on sensitive topics. *Western Journal of Nursing Research*, **10**(2), 163–179.

Coyle, A. (1998). Qualitative research in counselling psychology: using the counselling interview as a research instrument. In P. Clarkson (ed.), *Counselling Psychology: Integrating Theory, Research and Supervised Practice* (pp. 56–74). London: Routledge.

Coyle, A. & Wright, C. (1996). Using the counselling interview to collect research data on sensitive topics. *Journal of Health Psychology*, **1**(4), 431–440.

Crawford, J., Kippax, S., Onyx, J., Gault, U. & Benton, P. (1992). *Emotion and Gender: Constructing Meaning from Memory*. London: Sage Publications.

Cutcliffe, J.R. & Ramcharan, P. (2002). Leveling the playing field? Exploring the merits of ethics-as-process approach for judging qualitative research proposals. *Qualitative Health Research*, **12**(7), 1000–1010.

Daly, K. (1992). The fit between qualitative research and characteristics of families. In J.F. Gilgun, K. Day & G. Handel (eds.), *Qualitative Methods in Family Research* (pp. 3–11). Newbury Park: Sage Publications.

Daly, K. (2007). *Qualitative Methods for Family Studies and Human Development*. London: Sage Publications.

Dane, B. (2000). Child welfare workers: an innovative approach to interacting with secondary trauma. *Journal of Social Work Education*, **36**, 27–38.

Darlington, Y. & Scott, D. (2002). *Qualitative Research in Practice: Stories From the Field*. St. Leonards: Allen and Unwin.

Davis, H. (2001). The management of self: practical and emotional implications of ethnographic work in a public hospital setting. In K. Gilbert (ed.), *The Emotional Nature of Qualitative Research*. London: CRC Press.

De Raeve, L. (1994). Ethical issues in palliative care research. *Palliative Medicine*, **8**, 298–305.

Demi, A.S. & Warren, N.A. (1995). Issues in conducting sensitive research with vulnerable families. *Western Journal of Nursing Research*, **17**(2), 188–202.

Denzin, N. (1984). *On Understanding Emotion*. San Francisco: Josey Bass.

Denzin, N. (1989). *Interpretive Interactionism*. Newbury Park: Sage Publications.

Denzin, N. & Lincoln, Y.S. (eds.) (1994). *Handbook of Qualitative Research*. Thousand Oaks, CA: Sage Publications.

Denzin, N.K. & Lincoln, Y.S. (eds.) (2000). *Handbook of Qualitative Research* (2nd edn). Thousand Oaks, CA: Sage Publications.

Denzin, N.K. & Lincoln, Y.S. (2005a). *Handbook of Qualitative Research* (3rd edn). Thousand Oaks, CA: Sage Publications.

Denzin, N.K. & Lincoln, Y.S. (2005b). Introduction: the discipline and practice of qualitative research. In N.K. Denzin & Y.S. Lincoln (eds.), *Handbook of Qualitative Research* (3rd edn, pp.1–32). Thousand Oaks, CA: Sage Publications.

DeVault, M. (1997). Personal writing in social research: issues of production and interpretation. In R. Hertz (ed.), *Reflexivity and Voice* (pp.216–229). Thousand Oaks, CA: Sage Publications.

Dickson-Swift, V. (2000). *The Experience of Living with a Problem Gambler: Partners and Spouses Speak Out*. Unpublished Honours Thesis. Bendigo: La Trobe University.

Dickson-Swift, V. (2005). *Undertaking Sensitive Health Research: The Experiences of Researchers*. Bendigo: La Trobe University.

Dickson-Swift, V., James, E. & Kippen, S. (2005). Do university ethics committees adequately protect public health researchers? *Australian and New Zealand Journal of Public Health*, **29**(6), 576–582.

Dickson-Swift, V., James, E., Kippen, S. & Liamputtong, P. (2006). Blurring boundaries in qualitative health research on sensitive topics. *Qualitative Health Research*, **16**(6), 853–871.

Dickson-Swift, V., James, E.L., Kippen, S. & Liamputtong, P. (2007). Doing sensitive research: what challenges do qualitative researchers face? *Qualitative Research*, **7**(3), 327–353.

Dickson-Swift, V., James, E.L., Kippen, S. & Liamputtong, P. (2008). Risk to researchers in qualitative research on sensitive subjects: issues and strategies. *Qualitative Health Research*, **18**(1), 133–144.

Dickson-Swift, V., James, E.L., Kippen, S. & Liamputtong, P. (in press). Researching sensitive topics: qualitative research as emotion work. *Qualitative Research*.

Dollard, M. (2003). Introduction: context, theories and intervention. In M. Dollard, A.H. Winefield & H.R. Winefield (eds.), *Occupational Stress in the Service Professions* (pp.1–42). London: Taylor and Francis.

Draucker, C.B. (1999). The emotional impact of sexual violence research on participants. *Archives of Psychiatric Nursing*, **13**(4), 161–169.

Driscoll, T.R., Hull, B.P., Mandryk, J.A., Mitchell, R.A. & Howland, A.S. (1997). Minimizing the personal cost of involvement in research into traumatic death. *Safety Science*, **25**(1–3), 45–53.

Duncombe, J. & Jessop, J. (2002). 'Doing rapport' and the ethics of 'faking friendship'. In M. Mauthner, M. Birch, J. Jessop & T. Miller (eds.), *Ethics in Qualitative Research*. London: Sage Publications.

Dunn, L. (1991). Research alert! Qualitative research may be hazardous to your health! *Qualitative Health Research*, **1**(3), 388–392.

Dunscombe, J. & Marsden, D. (1996). Can we research the private sphere? Methodological and ethical problems in the study of the role of intimate emotion in personal relationships. In L. Morris & E.S. Lyon (eds.), *Gender Relations in Public and Private* (pp.140–153). Hampshire: MacMillan.

Dyregrov, K. (2004). Bereaved parents experience of research participation. *Social Science and Medicine*, **58**(2), 391–400.

Ellingson, L.L. (1998). 'Then you know how I feel': empathy, identification and reflexivity in fieldwork. *Qualitative Inquiry*, **4**(4), 492–514.

Ellis, C. (1991). Emotional sociology. *Studies in Symbolic Interaction*, **12**, 123–145.

Ellis, C. (1995). *Final Negotiations: A Story of Love, Loss and Chronic Illness*. Philadelphia, PA: Temple University Press.

Ellis, C. (2004). *The Ethnographic 'I': A Methodological Novel About Autoethnography*. Walnut Creek: AtlaMira Press.

Ellis, C. & Bochner, A. (eds.) (1996). *Composing Ethnography: Alternative Forms of Qualitative Writing*. Walnut Creek: AltaMira Press.

Ellis, C. & Bochner, A. (2000). Autoethnography, personal narrative, reflexivity: researcher as subject. In N.K. Denzin & Y.S. Lincoln (eds.), *Handbook of Qualitative Research* (2nd edn, pp.733–768). Thousand Oaks, CA: Sage Publications.

Ellis, C. & Bochner, P. (1999). Bringing emotion and personal narrative into medical social science. *Health*, **3**, 229–237.

Ellis, C., Kiesinger, C.E. & Tillmann-Healy, L.M. (1997). Interactive interviewing: talking about emotional experience. In R. Hertz (ed.), *Reflexivity and Voice* (pp.119–150). Thousand Oaks, CA: Sage Publications.

Ellsberg, M., Heise, L., Pena, R., Agurton, S. & Winkvist, A. (2001). Researching domestic violence against women: methodological and ethical considerations. *Studies in Family Planning*, **32**(1), 1–16.

Ely, M., Anzul, M., Friedman, T., Garner, D. & Steinmetz, A. (1991). *Doing Qualitative Research: Circles within Circles*. London: Falmer Press.

Emanuel, E.J., Wendler, D. & Grady, C. (2000). What makes clinical research ethical? *Journal of the American Medical Association*, **283**(20), 2701–2711.

England, P. (1992). *Comparable Worth: Theories and Evidence*. New York: Aldine.

Erlandson, D.A., Harris, E.L., Skipper, B. & Allen, S. (1993). *Doing Naturalistic Inquiry: A Guide to Methods*. Newbury Park: Sage Publications.

Etherington, K. (1996). The counsellor as researcher: boundary issues and critical dilemmas. *British Journal of Guidance and Counselling*, **24**(3), 339–346.

Etherington, K. (2007). Working with traumatic stories: from transcriber to witness. *International Journal of Social Research Methodology*, **10**(2), 85–97.

Faberow, N.L. (1963). *Taboo Topics*. New York: Atherton Press.

Ferguson, K. (2003). The impact of qualitative research on the researcher. *Paper presented at the Association for Qualitative Research Conference*. Coogee, Sydney.

Ferrell, J. & Hamm, M.S. (eds.) (1998). *Ethnography at the Edge: Crime, Deviance and Field Research*. Boston: Northeastern University Press.

Finch, J. (1984). It's great to have someone to talk to: the ethics and politics of interviewing women. In C. Bell & H. Roberts (eds.), *Social Researching: Politics, Problems, Practice* (pp.70–87). London: Routledge and Kegan Paul.

Fincham, B. (2006). Back to the 'old school': bicycle messengers employment and ethnography. *Qualitative Research*, **6**(2), 187–205.

Fineman, S. (1993). Organizations as emotional arenas. In S. Fineman (ed.), *Emotion in Organizations* (pp. 19–45). London: Sage Publications.

Flaskerud, J.H. & Winslow, B.J. (1998). Conceptualising vulnerable populations in health-related research. *Nursing Research*, **47**(2), 69–78.

Fonow, M.M. & Cook, J.A. (1991). Back to the future: a look at the second wave of feminist epistemology and methodology. In M.M. Fonow & J.A. Cook (eds.), *Beyond Methodology: Feminist Scholarship as Lived Research* (pp. 1–15). Indianna: Bloomington.

Fontana, A. & Frey, J. (1994). Interviewing: the art of science. In N. Denzin & Y. Lincoln (eds.), *Handbook of Qualitative Research* (pp. 361–376). London: Sage Publications.

Fox, N. (1998). 'Risks', hazards and life choices: reflections on health at work. *Sociology*, **32**(4), 665–687.

Fox, N. (1999). Postmodern reflections on 'risk', 'hazards' and life choices. In D. Lupton (ed.), *Risk and Sociocultural Theory: New Directions and Perspectives* (pp. 12–33). Cambridge: Cambridge University Press.

France, A., Bendelow, G. & Williams, S. (2000). A 'risky' business: researching the health beliefs of children and young people. In A. Lewis & G. Lindsay (eds.), *Researching the Health Beliefs of Children and Young People* (pp. 150–162). Buckingham: Open University Press.

Gadamer, H.G. (1995). *Truth and Method* (2nd rev. edn). New York: Continuum.

Gair, S. (2002). In the thick of it: a reflective tale from an Australian social worker/ qualitative researcher. *Qualitative Health Research*, **12**(1), 130–139.

Gale, J. (1992). When research interviews are more therapeutic than therapy interviews. *The Qualitative Report*, **1**(4). Available from http://www.nova.edu/ssss/QR/QR1-4/gale.html. [Accessed 31/3/2008].

Game, A. (1997). Sociology's emotions. *Canadian Review of Sociology and Anthropology*, **34**(4), 385–399.

Game, A. & Metcalfe, A. (1996). *Passionate Sociology*. London: Sage Publications.

Geertz, C. (1973). *The Interpretation of Culture*. New York: Basic Books.

Gergen, K. & Gergen, M. (1991). Towards reflexive methodologies. In F. Steir (ed.), *Research and Reflexivity* (pp. 77–95). Newbury Park, CA: Sage Publications.

Giddens, A. (1991). *Modernity and Self-Identity: Self and Society in the Late Modern Age*. Cambridge: Polity Press.

Giddens, A. (1992). *The Transformation on Intimacy*. Cambridge: Polity Press.

Giddens, A. (1993). *New Rules of Sociological Method: A Positive Critique of Interpretative Sociologies* (2nd edn). Cambridge: Polity Press.

Gilbert, K.R. (2001a). Introduction: why are we interested in emotions? In K.R. Gilbert (ed.), *The Emotional Nature of Qualitative Research* (pp. 3–15). London: CRC.

Gilbert, K.R. (2001b). Collateral damage? Indirect exposure of staff members to the emotions of qualitative research. In K.R. Gilbert (ed.), *The Emotional Nature of Qualitative Research* (pp. 147–161). London: CRC.

Gilligan, C. (1977). In a different voice: women's conceptions of self and or morality. *Harvard Educational Review*, **47**(4), 481–503.

Gilligan, C. (1982). *In a Different Voice: Psychological Theory and Women's Development*. Cambridge: Harvard University Press.

Glesne, C. & Peshkin, A. (1992). *Becoming Qualitative Researchers: An Introduction*. London: Longman.

Godwyn, M. (2006). Using emotional labor to create and maintain relationships using service interactions. *Symbolic Interactions*, **29**(4), 487–506.

Goffman, E. (1959). *The Presentation of Self in Everyday Life*. Harmondsworth, England: Penguin.

Goffman, E. (1973). The mortification of self. In R. Flacks (ed.), *Conformity, Resistance and Self-Determination* (pp. 66–92). Boston: Little, Brown and Co.

Goodrum, S. & Keys, J.L. (2007). Reflections on two studies of emotionally sensitive topics: bereavement from murder and abortion. *International Journal of Social Research Methodology*, **10**(4), 249–258.

Goodwin, D., Pope, C., Mort, M. & Smith, A. (2003). Ethics and ethnography: an experiential account. *Qualitative Health Research*, **13**(4), 567–577.

Grafanaki, S. (1996). How research can change the researcher? The need for sensitivity, flexibility and ethical boundaries in conducting qualitative research in counselling/ psychotherapy. *British Journal of Guidance and Counselling*, **24**(3), 329–338.

Grbich, C. (1999). *Qualitative Research in Health: An Introduction*. St Leonards: Allen and Unwin.

Grbich, C. (2007). *Qualitative Data Analysis: An Introduction*. London: Sage Publications.

Greater Vancouver Mental Health Service (1996). *Clinical Policy and Procedure Manual*. Vancouver, BC: Greater Vancouver Health Service.

Gregory, D., Russell, C.K. & Phillips, L.R. (1997). Beyond textual perfection: transcribers as vulnerable persons. *Qualitative Health Research*, **7**(2), 294–300.

Griffiths, S.P. (2003). Stress in psychological work. In M. Dollard, A.H. Winefield & H.R. Winefield (eds.), *Occupational Stress in the Service Professions* (pp. 359–388). London: Taylor and Francis.

Grinyer, A. (2004). The narrative correspondence method: what a follow-up study can tell us about the longer term effects on participants in emotionally demanding research. *Qualitative Health Research*, **14**(10), 1326–1341.

Grossman, F.K. & Kruger, L. (1999). Reflections on a feminist research project: subjectivity and the wish for intimacy and equality. *Psychology of Women Quarterly*, **23**, 117–135.

Guba, E.G. & Lincoln, Y.S. (1985). *Naturalistic Inquiry*. Newbury Park: Sage Publications.

Guba, E.G. & Lincoln, Y.S. (1994). Competing paradigms in qualitative research. In N.K. Denzin & Y.S. Lincoln (eds.), *Handbook of Qualitative Research* (pp. 105–117). Thousand Oaks, CA: Sage Publications.

Guba, E.G. & Lincoln, Y.S. (2005). Paradigmatic controversies, contradictions and emerging confluences. In N.K. Denzin & Y.S. Lincoln (eds.), *Handbook of Qualitative Research* (3rd edn, pp. 191–216). Thousand Oaks, CA: Sage Publications.

Habermas, Y. (1971). *Knowledge and Human Interests* (J.J. Shapiro, Trans.). Boston: Beacon Press.

Habermas, Y. (1988). *On the Logic of Social Sciences* (S.W. Nicholsen & J. Stark, Trans.). Oxford: Polity.

Hall, B.L. & Kuilg, J.C. (2004). Kanadier Mennonites: a case study examining research challenges amongst religious groups. *Qualitative Health Research*, **14**(3), 359–368.

Hammersley, M. & Atkinson, P. (1983). *Ethnography: Principles in Practice*. New York: Tavistock.

Harding, S. (1987). *Feminism and Methodology*. Bloomington: Indianna University Press.

Harding, S. (1991). *Whose Science? Whose Knowledge? Thinking from Women's Lives*. Buckingham: Open University Press.

Harris, J. & Huntington, A. (2001). Emotions as analytic tools: qualitative research, feelings, and psychotherapeutic insight. In K. Gilbert (ed.), *The Emotional Nature of Qualitative Research* (pp.129–145). London: CRC.

Harris, L.C. (2002). The emotional labour of barristers: an exploration of emotional labour by status professionals. *Journal of Management Studies*, **39**(4), 553–584.

Harrison, B. & Lyon, E.S. (1993). A note on ethical issues in the use of autobiography in sociological research. *Sociology*, **27**, 101–109.

Hart, N. & Wright-Crawford, A. (1999). Research as therapy, therapy as research: ethical dilemmas in new-paradigm research. *British Journal of Guidance and Counselling*, **27**(2), 205–214.

Hartmann, E. (1997). The concept of boundaries in counselling and psychotherapy. *British Journal of Guidance and Counselling*, **25**(2), 147–162.

Hayes, E.R., Carter, S.V., Carroll, M.C. & Morin, K.H. (1996). Managing fear associated with nursing in urban environments: first steps. *Public Health Nursing*, **13**(2), 90–96.

Heidegger, M. (1962). *Being and Time*. New York: Harper and Rowe.

Held, V. (1993). *Feminist Morality: Transforming Culture, Society and Politics*. Chicago: University of Chicago Press.

Hennings, J., Williams, J. & Haque, B.N. (1996). Exploring the health needs of Bangladeshi women: a case study in using qualitative research methods. *Health Education Journal*, **55**, 11–23.

Henslin, J.M. (2001). Studying deviance in four settings: research experiences with cabbies, suicides, drug users and abortionees. In A. Bryman (ed.), *Ethnography* (Vol. 2, pp.3–34). London: Sage Publications.

Hermansson, G. (1997). Boundaries and boundary management in counselling: the never-ending story. *British Journal of Guidance and Counselling*, **25**(2), 133–145.

Hertz, R. (1997). *Reflexivity and Voice*. Thousand Oaks, CA: Sage Publications.

Hess, R. (2006). Postabortion research: methodological and ethical issues. *Qualitative Health Research*, **16**(4), 580–587.

Hesse-Biber, S.N. & Leavy, L.P. (2005). *The Practice of Qualitative Research*. Thousand Oaks, CA: Sage Publications.

Hewitt, J. (2007). Ethical components of researcher–researched relationships in qualitative interviewing. *Qualitative Health Research*, **17**(8), 1149–1159.

Higgins, I. (1998). Reflections of conducting qualitative research with elderly people. *Qualitative Health Research*, **8**(6), 858–866.

Hochschild, A. (1979). Emotion work, feeling rules and social structure. *American Journal of Sociology*, **85**, 551–557.

Hochschild, A. (1983). *The Managed Heart: The Commercialization of Human Feeling*. Berkeley: University of California Press.

Hochschild, A. (1990). Ideology and emotion management: a perspective and path for future research. In T.D. Kemper (ed.), *Research Agendas in the Sociology of Emotions* (pp.117–142). New York: The University of New York Press.

Hochschild, A. (1998). The sociology of emotion as a way of seeing. In G. Bendelow & S.J. Williams (eds.), *Emotions in Social Life: Critical Themes and Contemporary Issues* (pp.3–15). London: Routledge.

Hoddinott, P. & Pill, R. (1997). Qualitative research interviewing by general practitioners. A personal view of the opportunities and pitfalls. *Family Practice,* **14**(4), 307–312.

Holland, J. (2007). Emotions and research. *International Journal of Social Research Methodology,* **10**(3), 195–209.

Hopkins, M. (1993). Is anonymity possible? Writing about refugees in the United States. In C. Brettel (ed.), *When They Read What We Write: The Politics of Ethnography* (pp. 62–90). Westport, CT: Bergin & Garvey.

Hubbard, G., Backett-Milburn, K. & Kemmer, D. (2001). Working with emotions: issues for the researcher in fieldwork and teamwork. *International Journal of Social Research Methodology,* **4**(2), 119–137.

Hughes, C. (1998). Learning to be intellectually insecure: the dis/empowering effects of reflexive practice. *International Journal of Social Research Methodology,* **1**, 281–296.

Husserl, E. (1970). *The Idea of Phenomenology.* The Hague, Netherlands: Martinus Nijhoff.

Hutchinson, S. & Wilson, H. (1994). Research and therapeutic interviews: a post-structuralist perspective. In J.M. Morse (ed.), *Critical Issues in Qualitative Research Methods.* Thousand Oaks, CA: Sage Publications.

Hutchinson, S.A., Wilson, M.E. & Wilson, H.S. (1994). Benefits of participating in research interviews. *IMAGE: Journal of Nursing Scholarship,* **26**(2), 161–164.

Israel, M. & Hay, I. (2006). *Research Ethics for Social Scientists: Between Ethical Conduct and Regulatory Compliance.* London: Sage Publications.

Jaggar, A. (1989). Love and knowledge: emotion in feminist epistemology. In A.R. Jaggar & S.R. Bordo (eds.), *Gender/Body/Knowledge* (pp. 145–171). New Brunswick: Rutgers University Press.

James, N. (1989). Emotional labour: skill and work in the social regulation of feelings. *Sociological Review,* **37**, 15–42.

James, N. (1992). Care = organisation + physical labor + emotional labor. *Sociology of Health and Illness,* **14**, 488–509.

James, N. (1993). Divisions of emotional labour: disclosure and anger. In S. Fineman (ed.), *Emotion in Organizations* (pp. 94–117). London: Sage Publications.

James, T. & Platzer, H. (1999). Ethical considerations in qualitative research with vulnerable groups: exploring lesbians and gay men's experiences of health care – a personal perspective. *Nursing Ethics,* **6**(1), 73–81.

Jamieson, J. (2000). Negotiating danger in fieldwork on crime. In G. Lee-Treweek & S. Linkogle (eds.), *Danger in the Field: Risk and Ethics in Social Research* (pp. 61–71). London: Routledge.

Jansen, G.G. & Davis, R. (1998). Honoring voice and visibility: sensitive topic research and feminist interpretive inquiry. *Affilia Journal of Women and Social Work,* **13**(3), 289–312.

Johnson, B. & Clarke, J. (2003). Collecting sensitive data: the impact on researchers. *Qualitative Health Research,* **13**(3), 421–434.

Johnson, B.M. & Plant, H. (1996). Collecting data from people with cancer and their families: what are the implications. In L. De Raeve (ed.), *Nursing Research: An Ethical and Legal Appraisal* (pp. 85–100). London: Bailliere Tindall.

Jones, S.H. (2005). Autoethnography: making the personal political. In N.K. Denzin & Y.S. Lincoln (eds.), *Handbook of Qualitative Research* (3rd edn, pp. 763–772). Thousand Oaks, CA: Sage Publications.

Katherine, A. (1991). *Boundaries: Where You End and I Begin*. New York: Simon and Schuster.

Kavanaugh, K. & Ayres, L. (1998). 'Not as bad as it could have been': Assessing and mitigating harm during research interviews on sensitive topics. *Research in Nursing and Health*, **21**, 91–97.

Kay, W. K. (2000). Role conflict and British Pentecostal ministers. *Journal of Psychology and Theology*, **28**, 119–125.

Kellehear, A. (1989). Ethics and social research. In J. Perry (ed.), *Doing Fieldwork: Eight Personal Accounts of Social Research* (pp. 64–80). Geelong: Deakin University Press.

Kellehear, A. (1990). *Dying of Cancer: The Final Year of Life*. London: Harvard Academic Publishers.

Kellehear, A. (1993a). Unobstrusive methods in medical practice. *Work-in-Progress Conference on Methodological Aspects of General Practice*. Canberra.

Kellehear, A. (1993b). Rethinking the survey. In D. Colquhoun & A. Kellehear (eds.), *Health Research in Practice: Political, Ethical and Methodological Issues* (pp. 126–137). London: Chapman Hall.

Kellehear, A. (1997). Unobtrusive methods in delicate situations. In J. Daly (ed.), *Ethical Intersections: Health Research, Methods and Researcher Responsibility*. Sydney: Allen & Unwin.

Kiesinger, C. (1998). From interview to story: writing 'Abbie's life'. *Qualitative Inquiry*, **4**(1), 71–96.

King, E. (1996). The use of self in qualitative research. In J. T. Richardson (ed.), *Handbook of Qualitative Research Methods for Psychology and Social Sciences* (pp. 175–189). Leicester: BPS Books.

Kitson, G. C., Clark, R. D., Rushforth, N. B. *et al.* (1996). Research on difficult family topics: helping new and experienced researchers cope with research on loss. *Family Relations*, **45**(2), 183–188.

Klein, R. D. (1983). How to do what we want to do: thoughts about feminist methodology. In G. Bowles & R. D. Klein (eds.), *Theories of Women's Studies* (pp. 88–104). Boston: Routledge and Keagan Paul.

Kleinman, S. (1991). Fieldworkers' feelings: what we felt, who we are, how we analyze. In W. B. Shaffir & R. A. Stebbins (eds.), *Experiencing Fieldwork: An Inside View of Qualitative Research* (pp. 184–195). Newbury Park: Sage Publications.

Kleinman, S. & Copp, M. A. (1993). *Emotions and Fieldwork*. Newbury Park: Sage Publications.

Kondora, L. L. (1993). A Heideggerian hermeneutical analysis of survivors of incest. *IMAGE: Journal of Nursing Scholarship*, **25**(1), 11–16.

Krieger, S. (1991). *Social Science and the Self: Personal Essays on an Art Form*. New Brunswick: Rutgers University Press.

Kvale, S. (1996). *InterViews: An Introduction to Qualitative Research Interviewing*. Thousand Oaks, CA: Sage Publications.

Lalor, J. G., Begley, C. M. & Devane, D. (2006). Exploring painful experiences: impact of emotional narratives on members of a qualitative research team. *Journal of Advanced Nursing*, **56**(6), 607–616.

Langford, D. R. (2000). Developing a safety protocol in qualitative research involving battered women. *Qualitative Health Research*, **10**(1), 113–142.

Lankshear, G. (2000). Bacteria and babies: a personal reflection on researcher risk in a hospital. In G. Lee-Treweek & S. Linkogle (eds.), *Danger in the Field: Risk and Ethics in Social Research* (pp.72–90). London: Routledge.

Lazarus, A.A. & Zur, O. (2002). *Dual Relationships and Psychotherapy* (Vol. 38). New York: Springer.

Lee-Treweek, G. (1996). Emotional work in care assistant work. In V. James & J. Gabe (eds.), *Health and the Sociology of Emotions.* Oxford: Blackwell.

Lee-Treweek, G. (2000). The insight of emotional danger: research experiences in a home for older people. In G. Lee-Treweek & S. Linkogle (eds.), *Danger in the Field: Risk and Ethics in Social Research* (pp.114–131). London: Routledge.

Lee-Treweek, G. & Linkogle, S. (eds.) (2000a). *Danger in the Field: Risk and Ethics in Social Research.* London: Routledge.

Lee-Treweek, G. & Linkogle, S. (2000b). Putting danger in the frame. In G. Lee-Treweek & S. Linkogle (eds.), *Danger in the Field: Risk and Ethics in Social Research* (pp.8–25). London: Routledge.

Lee, R.E., Eppler, C., Kendal, N. & Latty, C. (2001). Critical incidents in the professional lives of first MFT students. *Contemporary Family Therapy: An International Journal,* **23**, 51–61.

Lee, R.M. (1993). *Doing Research on Sensitive Topics.* London: Sage Publications.

Lee, R.M. (1995). *Dangerous Fieldwork.* Thousand Oaks, CA: Sage Publications.

Lee, R.M. & Renzetti, C. (1993). The problems of researching sensitive topics. In C.M. Renzetti & R.M. Lee (eds.), *Researching Sensitive Topics* (pp.3–12). Newbury Park: Sage Publications.

Leininger, M. (1981). The phenomenon of caring: importance, research questions and theoretical considerations. In M. Leininger (ed.), *Caring: An Essential Human Need* (pp.3–16). New Jersey: Charles B Slack.

Letherby, G. (2000). Dangerous liaisons: auto/biography in research and research writing. In G. Lee-Treweek & S. Linkogle (eds.), *Danger in the Field: Risk and Ethics in Social Research* (pp.91–113). London: Routledge.

Liamputtong, P. (2007). *Researching the Vulnerable: A Guide to Sensitive Research Methods.* London: Sage Publications.

Liamputtong, P. & Ezzy, D. (2005). *Qualitative Research Methods* (2nd edn). South Melbourne: Oxford University Press.

Liamputtong Rice, P. (1996). Health research and ethnic communities: reflections on practice. In D. Colquhoun & A. Kellehear (eds.), *Health Research in Practice* (Vol. 2). *Personal Experiences, Public Issues.* London: Chapman Hall.

Liamputtong Rice, P. (2000). *Hmong Women and Reproduction.* Westport: Bergin and Garvey.

Liamputtong Rice, P. & Ezzy, D. (1999). *Qualitative Research Methods: A Health Focus.* South Melbourne: Oxford University Press.

Lincoln, Y.S. & Guba, E.G. (1985). *Naturalistic Inquiry.* Beverly Hills: Sage Publications.

Lipson, J.G. (1994). Ethical issues in ethnography. In J.M. Morse (ed.), *Critical Issues in Qualitative Research Methods* (pp.332–355). Thousand Oaks, CA: Sage Publications.

Lipson, J.G. (1997). The politics of publishing: protecting participants confidentiality. In J.M. Morse (ed.), *Completing a Qualitative Project: Details and Dialogue* (pp. 39–61). Thousand Oaks, CA: Sage Publications.

Lipson, J.G. & Meleis, A. (1989). Methodological issues in research with immigrants. *Medical Anthropology*, **12**(1), 103–115.

Lofland, J. & Lofland, J. (1995). *Analyzing Social Settings: A Guide to Qualitative Observation and Analysis*. Belmont: Wadsworth Publishing.

Lonne, R. (2003). Social workers and human service practitioners. In M. Dollard, A.H. Winefield & H.R. Winefield (eds.), *Occupational Stress in the Service Professions* (pp.281–309). London: Taylor and Francis.

Lupton, D. (1994). *Medicine as Culture: Illness, Disease and the Body in Western Societies*. London: Sage Publications.

Lupton, D. (1995). *The Imperative of Health: Public Health and the Regulated Body*. London: Sage Publications.

Lupton, D. (1998). *The Emotional Self*. London: Sage Publications.

Lupton, D. (2002). 'Risk is part of your life': risk epistemologies among a group of Australians. *Sociology*, **36**(2), 317–334.

Malacrida, C. (2007). Reflexive journaling on emotional research topics: ethical issues for team researchers *Qualitative Health Research*, **17**(10), 1329–1339.

Maslach, C. (1982). *Burnout: The Cost of Caring*. Englewood Cliffs, NJ: Prentice Hall.

Maslach, C. (1998). A multidimensional theory of burnout. In C.L. Cooper (ed.), *Theories of Organisational Stress* (pp.68–85). Oxford: Oxford University Press.

Matocha, L.K. (1992). Case study interviews: caring for persons with AIDS. In J.F. Gilgun, K. Daly & G. Handel (eds.), *Qualitative Methods in Family Research* (pp. 66–84). Newbury Park: Sage Publications.

Mauthner, M., Birch, M., Jessop, J. & Miller, T. (eds.) (2002). *Ethics in Qualitative Research*. London: Sage Publications.

May, T. (1998). Reflexivity in the age of reconstructive social science. *International Journal of Social Research Methodology*, **1**, 7–24.

McCann, I.L. & Pearlman, L.A. (1990). Vicarious traumatization: a framework for understanding the psychological effects of working with victims. *Journal of Traumatic Stress Studies*, **3**, 131–149.

McCosker, H., Barnard, A. & Gerber, R. (2001). Undertaking sensitive research: issues and strategies for meeting the safety needs of all participants. *Forum: Qualitative Social Research [online journal]*. Available from http://qualitative-research.net/fqs/fqs-eng.htm [Accessed 20/12/2001].

McMahon, M. & Patton, W. (2002). *Supervision in the Helping Professions: A Practical Approach*. Sydney: Prentice Hall.

Meadows, L.M., Lagendyk, l. E., Thurston, W.E. & Eisener, A.C. (2003). Balancing culture, ethics and methods in qualitative health research with aboriginal peoples. *International Journal of Qualitative Methods*, **2**(4). Available from http://www.ualberta.ca/~iiqm/backissues/2_4/pdf/meadows.pdf [Accessed 9/10/2005].

Medical Research Council of Canada (MRC), National Science and Engineering Research Council of Canada (NSERC) & Social Science and Humanities Research Council of Canada (SSHRC) (1998). *Tri-Council Policy Statement: Ethical Conduct for Research Involving Humans*. Ottawa: MRC, NSERC, SSHRC.

Meerabeau, L. & Page, S. (1998). Getting the job done: emotions management and cardiopulmonary resuscitation in nursing. In G. Bendelow & S. Williams (eds.), *Emotions in Social Life* (pp.295–312). London: Routledge.

Melrose, M. (2002). Labour pains: some consideration on the difficulties of researching juvenile prostitution. *International Journal of Social Research Methodology*, **5**(4), 333–351.

Merleau-Ponty, M. (1962). *Phenomenology of Perception* (C. Smith, Trans.). New York: Routledge.

Mies, M. (1983). Toward a methodology for feminist research. In G. Bowles & R.D. Klein (eds.), *Theories of Women's Studies* (pp.117–139). Boston: Routledge and Keagan Paul.

Miller, J.M. & Tewksbury, R. (eds.) (2001). *Extreme Methods: Innovative Approaches to Social Science Research*. Boston, MA: Allyn and Bacon.

Miller, T. & Boulton, M. (2007). Changing constructions of informed consent: qualitative research and complex social worlds. *Social Science and Medicine*, **65**, 2199–2211.

Milling-Kinard, E. (1996). Conducting research on child maltreatment: effects on researchers. *Violence and Victims*, **11**(1), 65–69.

Minichiello, V., Madison, J., Hays, T., Courtney, M. & St. John, W. (1999). Qualitative interviews. In V. Minichiello, G. Sullivan, K. Greenwood & R. Axford (eds.), *Handbook for Research Methods in Health Sciences* (pp.395–417). Sydney: Addison-Wesley.

Minichiello, V., Aroni, R., Timewell, E. & Alexander, L. (2000). *In-Depth Interviewing* (2nd edn). Sydney: Longman.

Moran-Ellis, J. (1996). Close to home: the experience of researching child sexual abuse. In M. Hester, L. Kelly & J. Radford (eds.), *Women, Violence and Male Power* (pp.176–187). Buckingham: Open University.

Moreno, E. (1995). Rape in the field: reflections from a survivor. In D. Kulick & M. Wilson (eds.), *Taboo: Sex, Identity and Erotic Subjectivity in Anthropological Fieldwork* (pp.219–250). New York: Routledge.

Morgan, J.M. & Krone, K.J. (2001). Bending the rules of 'professional' display: emotional improvisation in caregiver performances. *Journal of Applied Communication Research*, **29**(4), 317–340.

Morley, L. (1996). Interrogating patriarchy: the challenges of feminist research. In V. Walsh & L. Morley (eds.), *Breaking Boundaries: Women in Higher Education* (pp.128–148). London: Taylor and Francis.

Morse, J.M. (ed.) (1997). *Completing a Qualitative Project: Details and Dialogue*. Thousand Oaks, CA: Sage Publications.

Morse, J.M. (2000). Researching illness and injury: methodological considerations. *Qualitative Health Research*, **10**(4), 538–546.

Morse, J.M. & Field, P.A. (1995). *Qualitative Research Methods for Health Professionals* (2nd edn). Thousand Oaks, CA: Sage Publications.

Morse, J.M., Solberg, S.M., Neander, W.L., Bottorff, J.L. & Johnson, J.L. (1990). Concepts of caring and caring as a concept. *Advances in Nursing Science*, **13**(1), 1–14.

Morse, J.M., Botorff, J., Neander, W. & Solberg, S. (1991). Comparative analysis of conceptualizations and theories of caring. *IMAGE: Journal of Nursing Scholarship*, **23**(2), 119–126.

Murray, B. (2003). Qualitative research interviews: therapeutic benefits for the participants. *Journal of Psychiatric and Mental Health Nursing*, **10**(2), 233–236.

Nespor, J. (2000). Anonymity and place in qualitative inquiry. *Qualitative Inquiry*, **6**(4), 546–569.

NHMRC (1995). *Ethical Aspects of Qualitative Methods in Health Research: An Information Paper for Institutional Ethics Committees.* Canberra: National Health and Medical Research Council.

NHMRC (1999). *National Statement on Ethical Conduct in Research Involving Humans.* Canberra: National Health and Medical Research Council.

NHMRC (2002). *Human Research Ethics Handbook: Commentary on the National Statement on Ethical Conduct in Research Involving Humans.* Canberra: National Health and Medical Research Council.

NHMRC (2007). *National Statement on Ethical Conduct in Human Research.* Canberra: National Health and Medical Research Council and Australian Vice Chancellors Committee.

Nias, J. (1996). Special issue: the emotions in teaching. *Cambridge Journal of Education,* **26**, 3.

Noddings, N. (1984). *Caring: A Feminine Approach to Ethics and Moral Education.* Berkeley, CA: University of California Press.

Noddings, N. (2003). *Caring: A Feminist Approach to Ethics and Moral Education* (2nd edn). Berkeley, CA: University of California Press.

Norris, J., Nurius, P.S. & Dimeff, L.A. (1996). Through her eyes: factors affecting women's perception of and resistance to acquaintances' sexual aggression threat. *Psychology of Women Quarterly,* **20**, 123–145.

Nurses Board of Victoria (2001). *Professional boundaries, Guidelines for Registered Nurses in Victoria.* Melbourne: Nurses Board of Victoria.

O'Brien, M. (1994). The managed heart revisited: health and social control. *Sociological Review,* **42**, 393–413.

O'Neill, M. (1996). Researching prostitution and violence: towards a feminist praxis. In M. Hester, L. Kelly & J. Radford (eds.), *Women, Violence and Male Power* (pp. 130–147). Buckingham: Open University.

Oakley, A. (1981). Interviewing women: a contradiction in terms. In H. Roberts (ed.), *Doing Feminist Research* (pp. 30–61). New York: Routledge.

Oakley, A. (1998). Gender, methodology and people's ways of knowing: some problems with feminism and the paradigm debate in social science. *Sociology,* **32**(4), 707–737.

Olesen, V. (2005). Early millennial feminist qualitative research: challenges and contours. In N.K. Denzin & Y.S. Lincoln (eds.), *Handbook of Qualitative Research* (3rd edn, pp. 235–278). Thousand Oaks, CA: Sage Publications.

Orb, A., Eisenhauer, L. & Wynaden, D. (2001). Ethics in qualitative research. *Journal of Nursing Scholarship,* **33**(11), 93–104.

Owens, D. (1996). Men, emotions and the research process: the role of interviews in sensitive areas. In K. Carter & S. Delamount (eds.), *Qualitative Research: The Emotional Dimension* (pp. 56–65). Aldershot: Averbury.

Paradis, E.K. (2000). Feminist and community psychology ethics in research with homeless women. *American Journal of Community Psychology,* **28**(6), 839–858.

Parker, B. & Ulrich, Y. (1990). A protocol of safety: research on abuse of women. *Nursing Research,* **39**(4), 248–250.

Parris, D., Du Mont, J. & Gombay, B. (2005). Co-operation or co-optation? Assessing the methodological benefits and barriers involved in conducting qualitative research through medical institutional settings. *Qualitative Health Research,* **15**(5), 686–697.

Patai, D. (1991). US academics and third world women: is ethical research possible? In S. Gluck & D. Patai (eds.), *Women's Words: The Feminist Practice of Oral History* (pp. 136–150). London: Routledge.

Paterson, B.L., Gregory, D. & Thorne, S. (1999). A protocol for researcher safety. *Qualitative Health Research*, **9**(2), 259–269.

Patton, M.Q. (1990). *Qualitative Evaluation and Research Methods* (2nd edn). Newbury Park: Sage Publications.

Payne, S. (1994). Issues for researchers using qualitative methods. *Health Psychology Update*, **16**, 7–9.

Pearlman, L.A. (1995). Self-care for trauma therapists: ameliorating vicarious traumatization. In B. Stamm Hundall (ed.), *Secondary Traumatic Stress: Self-care Issues for Clinicians, Researchers and Educators* (pp. 52–64). Lutherville: Sidran Press.

Pennebaker, J.W. (1990). *Opening Up: The Healing Power of Expressing Emotions*. New York: The Guildford Press.

Perry, J. (1989). *Doing Fieldwork: Eight Personal Accounts of Social Research*. Geelong: Deakin University Press.

Petronio, S. (1991). Communication boundary management: a theoretical model of managing disclosure of private information between marital couples. *Communication Theory*, **1**, 311–335.

Pierce, J.L. (1999). Emotional labor among paralegals. *Annals of the American Academy of Political and Social Science*, **561**, 127–142.

Platzer, H. & James, T. (1997). Methodological issues in conducting sensitive research on lesbian and gay men's experience of nursing care. *Journal of Advanced Nursing*, **25**(3), 626–633.

Pyett, P. (2001). Innovation and compromise: responsibility and reflexivity in research and vulnerable groups. In J. Daly, M. Guillemin & S. Hill (eds.), *Technologies and Health: Critical Compromises*. Melbourne: Oxford University Press.

Rager, K.B. (2005a). Compassion stress and the qualitative researcher. *Qualitative Health Research*, **15**(3), 423–430.

Rager, K.B. (2005b). Self-care and the qualitative researcher: when collecting data can break your heart. *Educational Researcher*, **34**(4), 23–27.

Ramos, M.C. (1989). Some ethical implications of qualitative research. *Research in Nursing and Health*, **12**, 57–63.

Reinharz, S. (1992). *Feminist Methods in Social Research*. New York: Oxford University Press.

Reinharz, S. (1997). Who am I? The need for a variety of selves in the field. In R. Hertz (ed.) *Reflexivity and Voice* (pp. 3–20). Thousand Oaks, CA: Sage Publications.

Renzetti, C. & Lee, R.M. (eds.) (1993). *Researching Sensitive Topics*. Newbury Park: Sage Publications.

Ribbens, J. & Edwards, R. (1998). *Feminist Dilemmas in Qualitative Research: Public Knowledge and Private Lives*. London: Sage Publications.

Richards, H.M. & Schwartz, L.J. (2002). Ethics of qualitative research: are there special issues for health services research? *Family Practice*, **19**(2), 135–139.

Richardson, L. (1994). Writing: a method of inquiry. In N.K. Denzin & Y.S. Lincoln (eds.), *Handbook of Qualitative Research* (pp. 516–529). Thousand Oaks, CA: Sage Publications.

Richardson, L. (1997). *Fields of Play: Constructing an Academic Life*. New Brunswick: Rutgers.

Richardson, L. & Lockeridge, E. (2004). *Travels With Ernest: Crossing the Literary/ Sociological Divide*. Walnut Creek: AltaMira Press.

Richardson, L. & St Pierre, E.D. (2005). Writing: a method on inquiry. In N.K. Denzin & Y.S. Lincoln (eds.), *Handbook of Qualitative Research* (3rd edn, pp.959–978). Thousand Oaks, CA: Sage Publications.

Rickard, W. (2003). Collaboration with sex workers in oral history. *The Oral History Review*, 30(1), 47–59.

Ridge, D., Hee, A. & Aroni, R. (1999). Being 'real' in suicide prevention evaluation: the role of the ethnographers emotions under traumatic conditions. *Australian Journal of Primary Health-Interchange*, 5(3), 21–31.

Ringheim, K. (1995). Ethical issues in social science research with special reference to sexual behaviour research. *Social Science and Medicine*, 40(12), 1691–1697.

Roach, M.S. (1987). *The Human Act of Caring: A Blueprint for Health Professionals*. Toronto: Canadian Hospital Association.

Roberts, B. (2007). *Getting The Most Out Of The Research Experience: What Every Researcher Needs To Know*. Los Angeles, CA: Sage Publications.

Roberts, J.M. & Saunders, T. (2005). Before, during and after: realism, reflexivity and ethnography. *Sociological Review*, 53(2), 294–313.

Robertson, J. (2000). Ethical issues and researching sensitive topics: mature women and bulimia. *Feminism and Psychology*, 10(4), 531–537.

Rogers, J.K. (1995). Just a temp: experience and structure of alienation in temporary clerical employment. *Work and Occupation*, 22, 137–166.

Ronai, C.R. (1995). Multiple reflection of child sexual abuse: an argument for a layered account. *Journal of Contemporary Ethnography*, 23, 395–426.

Ronai, C.R. (1996). My mother is mentally retarded. In C. Ellis & A. Bochner (eds.), *Composing Ethnography: Alternative Forms of Qualitative Writing* (pp.109–131). Walnut Creek: AltaMira Press.

Ronai, C.R. & Ellis, C. (2001). Turn-ons for money: international strategies of the table dancer. In J.M. Miller & R. Tewksbury (eds.), *Extreme Methods: Innovative Approaches to Social Science Research* (pp.168–182). Boston: Allen & Unwin.

Rosaldo, M. (1984). Toward an anthropology of self and feeling. In R.A. Shweder & R.A. Levine (eds.), *Culture Theory: Essays on Mind, Self and Emotion* (pp.137–157). Cambridge: Cambridge University Press.

Rosenblatt, P.C. (1995). Ethics of qualitative interviewing with grieving families. *Death Studies*, 19, 139–155.

Rosenblatt, P.C. (2001). Qualitative research as a spiritual experience. In K. Gilbert (ed.), *The Emotional Nature of Qualitative Research* (pp.111–128). London: CRC.

Rosenblatt, P.C. & Fischer, L.R. (1993). Qualitative family research. In P.G. Boss, W.J. Doherty, R. LaRossa, W.R. Schumm & S.K. Steinmetz (eds.), *Sourcebook of Family Theories and Methods: A Contextual Approach* (pp.167–177). New York: Plenum.

Rowling, L. (1999). Being in, being out, being with: affect and the role of the qualitative researcher in loss and grief research. *Mortality*, 4(2), 167–181.

Russell, C. (1999). Interviewing vulnerable old people: ethical and methodological implications of imagining our subjects. *Journal of Ageing Studies*, 13(4), 403–427.

Ruthman, J., Jackson, J., McClusky, M. *et al.* (2004). Using clinical journaling to capture critical thinking across the curriculum. *Nursing Education Perspectives*, **25**, 120–123.

Sampson, H. & Thomas, M. (2003). Lone researchers at sea: gender, risk and responsibility. *Qualitative Research*, **3**(2), 165–189.

Sandelowski, M. (1994). Notes on transcription. *Research in Nursing and Health*, **17**, 311–314.

Scarce, R. (1994). (No) trial (but) tribulations: when courts and ethnography conflict. *Journal of Contemporary Ethnography*, **23**(2), 123–149.

Schauben, L.J. & Frazier, P.A. (1995). Vicarious trauma: the effects on female counsellors of working with sexual violence survivors. *Psychology of Women Quarterly*, **19**, 49–64.

Schramm, K. (2005). You have your history. Keep your hands off ours: on being rejected in the field. *Social Anthropology*, **13**, 171–183.

Scopelliti, J., Judd, F., Grigg, M. *et al.* (2004). Dual relationships in mental health practice: issues for clinicians in rural settings. *Australian and New Zealand Journal of Psychiatry*, **38**, 953–959.

Scott, S. (1998). Here be dragons: researching the unbelievable, hearing the unthinkable. A feminist sociologist in uncharted territory. *Sociological Research Online*, **3**(3).

Sexton, L. (1999). Vicarious traumatisation of counsellors and effects on workplaces. *British Journal of Guidance and Counselling*, **27**, 393–403.

Seymour, J., Bellamy, G., Gott, M., Ahmedzai, S.H. & Clark, D. (2002). Using focus groups to explore older people's attitudes to end of life care. *Ageing and Society*, **22**, 517–526.

Shaffir, W.B. & Stebbins, R.A. (eds.) (1991). *Experiencing Fieldwork: An Inside View of Qualitative Research.* Newbury Park: Sage Publications.

Shaffir, W.B., Stebbins, R.A. & Turowetz, A. (eds.) (1980). *Fieldwork Experience: Qualitative Approaches to Social Research.* New York: St. Martins Press.

Sharma, U. & Black, P. (2001). Look good, feel better: beauty therapy as emotional labour. *Sociology*, **35**(4), 913–919.

Sieber, J.E. (1992). *Planning Ethically Responsible Research.* Newbury Park: Sage Publications.

Sieber, J.E. (1993). The ethics and politics of sensitive research. In C. Renzetti & R. Lee (eds.), *Researching Sensitive Topics* (pp. 14–26). Newbury Park: Sage Publications.

Sieber, J.E. & Stanley, B. (1988). Ethical and professional dimensions of socially sensitive research. *American Psychologist*, **43**, 49–55.

Sin, C.H. (2005). Seeking informed consent: reflection on research practice. *Sociology*, **39**(2), 277–294.

Small, E. (1995). Valuing the unseen emotional labour of nursing. *Nursing Times*, **91**(26), 40–41.

Smith, A.C. & Kleinman, S. (1989). Managing emotions in medical school: students contacts with the living and the dead. *Social Psychology Quarterly*, **52**, 56–69.

Smith, D.E. (1987). *The Everyday World as Problematic: A Feminist Sociology.* Boston: Northeastern University Press.

Smith, L. (1992). Ethical issues in interviewing. *Journal of Advanced Nursing*, **17**, 98–103.

Smith, P. (1991). The nursing process: raising the profile of emotional care in nurse training. *Journal of Advanced Nursing*, **16**, 74–81.

Smith, P. (1992). *The Emotional Labour of Nursing*. Basingstoke: Macmillan.

Social Research Association (2006). *A Code of Practice for the Safety of Social Researchers*. Available from http://www.the-sra.org.uk/documents/word/safety_code_of_practice.doc [Accessed 19/09/2007].

Socolar, R., Runyan, D.K. & Amata-Jackson, L. (1995). Methodological and ethical issues related to studying child maltreatment. *Journal of Family Issues*, **16**, 565–586.

Spalek, B. (2007). A critical reflection on researching black Muslim women's lives post-September 11th. *International Journal of Social Research Methodology*, **8**(5), 405–418.

Sque, M. (2000). Researching the bereaved: an investigators experience. *Nursing Ethics*, **7**(1), 23–33.

Stacey, J. (1988). Can there be a feminist ethnography? *Women's Studies International Forum*, **11**(1), 21–27.

Stanko, E.A. (1997). 'I second that emotion'. Reflections on feminism, emotionality and research on sexual violence. In M.D. Schwartz (ed.), *Researching Sexual Violence Against Women: Methodological and Personal Perspectives* (pp.74–85). Thousand Oaks, CA: Sage Publications.

Stanley, B., Stanley, M., Lautin, A., Kane, J. & Schwartz, N. (1981). Preliminary findings on psychiatric patients as research participants: a population risk? *American Journal of Psychiatry*, **138**, 669–671.

Stanley, L. (ed.) (1990). *Feminist Praxis: Research, Theory and Epistemology*. London: Routledge.

Stanley, L. & Wise, S. (1983). *Breaking Out: Feminist Consciousness and Feminist Research*. London: Routledge and Kegan Paul.

Stanley, L. & Wise, S. (1990). Method, methodology and epistemology in the feminist research process. In L. Stanley (ed.), *Feminist Praxis, Research, Theory and Epistemology in Feminist Sociology*. London: Routledge.

Stanley, L. & Wise, S. (1991). Feminist research, feminist consciousness and experiences of sexism. In M.M. Fonow & J. Cook (eds.), *Beyond Methodology: Feminist Scholarship as Lived Research* (pp.266–291). Bloomington: Indianna University Press.

Stanley, L. & Wise, S. (1993). *Breaking Out Again: Feminist Consciousness and Feminist Research* (2nd edn). London: Routledge and Kegan Paul.

Stebbins, R.A. (1991). Do we ever leave the field? In W.B. Shaffir & R.A. Stebbins (eds.), *Experiencing Fieldwork: An Inside View of Qualitative Research* (pp.248–255). Newbury Park: Sage Publications.

Steinberg, A.M., Pynoos, R.S., Goenjaan, A.K., Sossanabadi, H. & Sherr, L. (1999). Are researchers bound by child abuse reporting laws? *Violence and Victims*, **5**(1), 67–71.

Steinberg, R.L. & Figart, D.M. (1999). Emotional labor since 'The Managed Heart'. *Annals of the American Academy of Political and Social Science*, **561**, 8–26.

Stoler, L.R. (2002). Researching childhood sexual abuse: anticipating effects on the researcher. *Feminism and Psychology*, **12**(2), 269–274.

Sullivan, K. (1998). Managing the 'sensitive' interview: a personal account. *Nurse Researcher*, **6**(2), 72–85.

Swanson, K.M. (1999). Research-based practice with women who have had miscarriages. *IMAGE: Journal of Nursing Scholarship*, **31**(4), 339–345.

Taylor, S. & Bogdan, R. (1998). *Introduction to Qualitative Research Methods: A Guidebook and Resource* (3rd edn). New York: Wiley.

Taylor, W.K., Magnussen, L. & Amundson, M.J. (2001). The lived experience of battered women. *Violence Against Women*, **7**(5), 563–585.

Tee, S.R. & Lathlean, J.A. (2004). The ethics of conducting a co-operative inquiry with vulnerable people. *Journal of Advanced Nursing*, **47**(5), 536–543.

Thoits, P.A. (1990). Emotional deviance: research agenda. In T.D. Kemper (ed.), *Research Agendas in the Sociology of Emotions* (pp. 180–203). New York: University of New York Press.

Tillman, L.C. (2003). Mentoring, reflection and reciprocal journaling. *Theory Into Practice*, **42**, 226–233.

Tolich, M.B. (1993). Alienating and liberating emotions at work: supermarket clerks' performance of customer service. *Journal of Contemporary Ethnography*, **22**, 361–381.

Turner, B. (1992). *Regulating Bodies: Essays in Medical Sociology*. New York: Routledge.

Usher, K. & Holmes, C. (1997). Ethical aspects of phenomenological research with mentally ill people. *Nursing Ethics*, **4**(1), 49–56.

Van Hooft, S. (1995). *Caring: An Essay in the Philosophy of Ethics*. Colorado: University Press of Colorado.

Van Maanen, J. (1988). *Tales of the Field: On Writing Ethnography*. Chicago: Chicago Press.

Van Maanen, J. (1990a). *Researching Lived Experience*. Ontario: University of Western Ontario.

Van Maanen, J. (1990b). The smile factory work at Disneyland. In P.J. Frost, L.F. Louis, C.C. Lundberg & J. Martin (eds.), *Reframing Organizational Culture* (pp. 58–76). Newbury Park: Sage Publications.

Van Maanen, J. & Kunda, G. (1989). 'Real feelings': emotional expressions and organizational culture. In B.M. Straw & L.L. Cummings (eds.), *Research in Organizational Behaviour* (Vol. 11). Greenwich, CT: JAI Press.

Volker, D.L. (2004). Methodological issues associated with studying an illegal act. *Advances in Nursing Science*, **27**(2), 117–128.

Waldrop, D. (2004). Ethical issues in qualitative research with high-risk populations: handle with care. In D.K. Padgett (ed.), *The Qualitative Research Experience* (pp. 236–249). Belmont, CA: Wadsworth.

Walker, R. & Clark, J.J. (1999). Heading off boundary problems: clinical supervision as risk management. *Psychiatric Services*, **50**(11), 1435–1439.

Warr, D. (2004). Stories in the flesh and voices in the head: reflections on the context and impact of research with disadvantaged populations. *Qualitative Health Research*, **14**(4), 578–587.

Warren, C. (2002). Qualitative interviewing. In J.F. Gubrium & J.A. Holstein (eds.), *Handbook of Interview Research: Context & Method* (pp. 83–102). Thousand Oaks, CA: Sage Publications.

Watson, L., Irwin, J. & Michalske, S. (1991). Researcher as friend: methods of the interviewer in a longitudinal study. *Qualitative Health Research*, **1**(4), 497–514.

Wax, R. (1971). *Doing Fieldwork: Warnings and Advice*. Chicago: University of Chicago Press.

Webb, S.B. (1997). Training for maintaining appropriate boundaries in counselling. *British Journal of Guidance and Counselling*, **25**(2), 175–188.

Weber, M. (ed.) (1949). *The Methodology of the Social Sciences*. Glencoe III: Free Press.

Weber, S. (1986). The nature of interviewing. *Phenomenology & Pedagogy*, **4**(2), 65–72.

Wenger, C. (2002). Interviewing older people. In J.F. Gubrium & J.A. Holstein (eds.), *Handbook of Interview Research: Context and Method* (pp. 259–278). Thousand Oaks, CA: Sage Publications.

Wharton, A.S. (1993). The affective consequences of service work. *Work and Occupations*, **20**, 205–232.

Wharton, A.S. (1999). The psychosocial consequences of emotional labor. *Annals of the American Academy of Political and Social Science*, **561**, 158–176.

Wharton, A.S. & Erickson, R.J. (1993). Managing emotions on the job and at home: understanding the consequences of multiple emotional roles. *Academy of Management Review*, **18**(3), 457–486.

Wichroski, M.A. (1994). The secretary: invisible labour in the workworld of women. *Human Organization*, **53**, 33–41.

Wilkins, R. (1993). Taking it personally: a note on emotion and autobiography. *Sociology*, **27**(1), 93–101.

Williams, S. (1998). Modernity and the emotions: corporeal reflections on the (ir)rational. *Sociology*, **32**, 121–139.

Williams, S.J. & Bendelow, G. (1998). *The Lived Body: Sociological Themes, Embodied Issues*. New York: Routledge.

Willis, J.W. (2007). *Foundations of Qualitative Research: Interpretive and Critical Approaches*. London: Sage Publications.

Wincup, E. (2001). Feminist research with women awaiting trial: the effects of participants in the qualitative research process. In K. Gilbert (ed.), *The Emotional Nature of Qualitative Research* (pp. 17–35). London: CRC.

Wray, N., Markovic, M. & Manderson, L. (2007). 'Researcher saturation': the impact of data triangulation and intensive-research practices on the research and qualitative research process. *Qualitative Health Research*, **17**(10), 1392–1402.

Young, E.H. & Lee, R.M. (1996). Fieldworker feelings as data: 'emotion work' and 'feeling rules' in first person accounts of sociological fieldwork. In V. James & J. Gabe (eds.), *Health and Sociology of Emotions*. Oxford: Blackwell Publishers Ltd.

Zapf, D., Seifert, C., Schmutte, B., Mertini, H. & Holz, M. (2001). Emotion work and job stressors and their effects on burnout. *Psychology and Health*, **16**, 527–545.

Index